Blood Testing

Results and Analysis

ESSENTIAL VITAMINS,
MINERALS AND SUPPORTING
FOODS

Sidney Krimsky

ISBN: 979-8-3303-9105-9 (sc)
ISBN: 979-8-3304-0079-9 (hc)
ISBN: 979-8-3303-9255-1 (e)

THE EWINGS PUBLISHING

One Galleria Blvd., Suite 1900, Metairie,
LA 70001 1-888-421-2397

Compiled from Medical Sources by Sidney Krimsky

B.S., M.S.M.E., MBA, P.E.

Blood Test Results, Essential Vitamins and Minerals from Foods

This book is not a medical textbook. It is a primer for patients who want to know more about the results of their blood tests, and the essential vitamins and minerals found in foods. The results of blood tests may be used as a predictor of co-morbidities (multiple illnesses at the same time).

This book is a study of the blood test results and the desired ranges of the measurements. The consequences of measurements that fall below or above the desired range are presented from data taken from the testing agencies and the Mayo Clinic. Measurements falling outside the desired range may have medical consequences. This booklet does not replace medical analysis or advice by a physician but adds to the patient's understanding of the blood test measurements. The blood tests are performed to evaluate the health of the liver, lungs, heart, thyroid, prostate, and immune system. There are three components to a diagnosis: 1) science employing measurements, X-Rays, sonograms, blood tests, urine tests, stool tests, etc. 2) evaluation of test results by a physician using his or her experience, and
3) the preference of the patients.

Measurements falling outside the desired range have to be evaluated by a physician, who can decide

1) to do nothing
2) to recommend a re-test
3) to recommend medication
4) to write a prescription
5) to send the patient to a specialist

Trace minerals and vitamins and essential foods are listed. A summary of "desired ranges" from several testing labs are compared listed at the end of the booklet.

A large number of laboratory Blood tests are widely available. Many Blood tests are specialized to focus on a particular disease or group of diseases. Many different Blood tests are used commonly in many specialties and in general practice.

What is a Blood test? Blood tests are an essential diagnostic tool. Blood is made up of different kinds of cells and contains other compounds, including various salts and certain proteins. Blood tests reveal details about these blood cells, blood compounds, salts and proteins

The liquid portion of the tested blood is plasma. When our blood clots outside the body, the blood cells and some of the proteins in blood turn into a solid. The remaining liquid is called serum, which can be used in chemical tests and in other Blood tests to find out how the immune system fights diseases. Doctors take blood samples and grow the organisms, found in blood tests, that cause illness, to evaluate each, microscopically.

Since most blood test reference ranges (often referred to as 'normal' ranges of blood test results) are typically defined as the range of values of the median 95% of the healthy population, it is unlikely that a given blood sample, even from a healthy patient, will show "normal" values for every blood test taken. Therefore, caution should be exercised to prevent overreaction to mild abnormalities without the interpretation of those tests by your examining physician. Again, a blood test, though important, is only a part of the final diagnosis of a health problem.

Physicians rely on "Blood-work," or clinical laboratory diagnostic blood testing to diagnose medical conditions. From this blood testing the medical professional then prescribes therapies and remedies, based on those blood tests. Blood test results reveal blood disorders and also rare blood types. Good blood tests make possible state-of-the-art lab procedures that can be provided directly to the public in private and these blood tests can be provided affordably.

How is a Blood test performed? Blood samples taken for Blood testing can be taken either from an artery or a vein. A few drops of blood are needed, most of the time. It is often enough to take a small drop from the tip of your finger and then squeeze the blood out for blood testing. Most blood tests taken from an artery (arteries carry fresh, oxygenated blood from the heart) most often from those arteries near the elbow. First a tourniquet is tied around the upper arm to make the artery easy to find and take the blood for the blood test.

The place where the injection is to take place is then made sterile and then a hollow needle is put into the artery. The needle will be attached either to a blood test sample bottle or to a syringe where the plunger is pulled back to create low negative pressure. When the needed amount of Blood for testing has been removed from the artery, the needle is removed. The area is then re-cleaned and pressure is placed on the area with a small ball of cotton. This is pressed against the area for a couple of minutes before applying a bandage. Blood test results are important in Blood disorders and with rare blood types. Blood tests are relatively painless. Some of the most common blood tests are as follows:

Allergy Blood Testing
Blood Tests for
Autoimmune Diseases
Blood Diseases Testing
Cancer Detection Blood
Testing Blood
Cholesterol Test
Diabetes Blood Tests
DNA, Paternity and Genetic
Testing Blood Tests for
Drug Screening
Environmental Toxin Blood

Testing Fitness, Nutrition
and Anti-Aging
Gastrointestinal Diseases Revealed by Blood Tests
Blood Testing for Heart
Health Hormones and Metabolism
Infectious Disease Blood Tests
Kidney Disease Blood Test Liver
Diseases Blood Testing
Sexually Transmitted Diseases (STD's)
Blood Tests Thyroid Disease Blood
Tests

Screening Blood tests are used to try to detect a disease when there is little or no evidence that a person has a suspected disease. For example, measuring cholesterol levels helps to identify one of the risks of heart disease. These screening tests are performed on people who may show no symptoms of heart disease, as a tool for the physician to detect a potentially harmful and evolving condition. In order for screening tests to be the most useful they must be readily available, accurate, inexpensive, pose little risk, and cause little discomfort to the patient.

Diagnostic Blood tests are utilized when a specific disease is suspected to verify the presence and the severity of that disease, including allergies, HIV, AIDS, Hepatitis, cancer, Covid, etc.

Platelet testing is a blood test that is often used by doctors. Platelets are very small cells in the Blood. These clump together at places where injurys occur to blood vessels. Platelets are the basis of the blood clot that normally forms when the skin is broken.

A blood test revealing a low platelet count can make us vulnerable to bleeding, sometimes even without an injury. Some of the causes of a low blood platelet count include autoimmune diseases, where the effected individual produces an antibody to his or her own platelets, chemotherapy, leukemia, viral infections and some medicines. High numbers of platelets make an individual more vulnerable to blood clotting. High Blood platelet counts are always found where a condition involving bone marrow such as leukemia, cancer and other blood borne conditions that are revealed by blood test results. No blood test is completely accurate all of the time. Sometimes a test result is incorrectly abnormal in a person who does not have the suspected disease (a false-positive result). Sometimes a test result is incorrectly normal in a person who has the disease (a false-negative result). Tests are rated in terms of their sensitivity (the probability that their Blood testing results will be positive when a disease is present) and their specificity (the probability that their test results will be negative when a disease is not present). A very sensitive test is unlikely to miss the disease in people who have it, however, it may falsely indicate disease in healthy people. Blood test results are important in blood disorders and with rare blood types. A very specific test is unlikely to indicate disease in healthy people. Although, it may miss the disease in some who have it. Problems with sensitivity and specificity can be largely overcome by using several different blood tests.

Because your physician can not always be sure whether or not the reported result of a particular test from a particular person is false or true, a person with an abnormal result may often need to be re-tested or undergo a different type of testing. Links to Free population

Normal test result values are expressed as a reference range, which is based on the average values in a healthy population; 95% of healthy people have values within this range. These values vary somewhat among laboratories, due to methodology and even geography. Blood tests and Blood testing methods and quality vary widely in different parts of the world and in different parts of many countries, due to characteristics in the racial blood differences and ethnic blood characteristics, among other factors.

American Blood laboratories use a different version of the metric system than does most of the rest of the world, which uses the Systeme Internationale (SI). In some cases translation between the two systems is easy, but the difference between the two is most pronounced in the measu measurement of chemical concentration. The American system generally uses mass per unit volume, while SI uses moles per unit volume. Since Mass p mass volume varies with the molecular weight of the substance being analyzed, conversion between American and SI units requires many different .differt conversion factors. A mol equals 1.0 when the molecular weight equals the weight in grams, ie. 32 grams of oxygen = 1 mol. Mol is short for molecule.

Doctors recommend periodical Personal Blood Testing. Your personal norms must be considered over time. Each individual has his or her own unique personal Blood test normal range.

The results of virtually all blood tests are compared to “normal ranges” as provided on a “Lab Results Report.” If your tests indicate that you are within within the normal range, you are most often considered normal. A “normal” Blood test result does not necessarily mean that you are healthy.

Sources:

Enzo Clinical Labs and Quest Diagnostics

Wikipedia

Dr. Marc Mccosi, PhD

Unsourced Ranges on the Internet

Merriam Webster's Dictionary

Reference Guide for Nursing, Jill E. Winland-Brown, EdD, MSM, ARNP

Mayo Clinic

Dimensions of measurements pages 62-68

mL	milliter
mg	milligrams
picograms	10^{-9} grams
g/ml	grams/milliter
micrograms	10^{-6} grams
cells/milliter	
nmol/liter	nanograms/ atomic weight per liter

COMPLETE BLOOD TEST RESULTS, DISEASES, AND ESSENTIAL VITAMINS, MINERALS & FOODS

CHAPTER 1

Comprehensive Metabolic Panel

Name	Meaning	Descriptor/What it does	High	Low
Glucose	Simple Sugar	$C_6H_{12}O_6$/provides energy to body makes cellulose for cell walls	Hyperglycemia (too much sugar) nausea, vomiting, abdominal pain, shortness of breath, diabetes poor wound healing	Hypoglycemia: (too little sugar loss of energy)
BUN	Blood Urea Nitrogen	Measures BUN in blood	Kidneys not working well, urinary tract, Infection, recent heart attack, congestive heart failure	Low protein diet, hunger malnutrition, liver disease, dehydration, gastrointestinal Bleeding, not enough blood flow to Kidneys
Creatinine	Creatinine is a waste product	Filtered by kidneys	Acute kidney failure anemia and small kidney size	Chronic kidney failure
eGFR	Estimated Glomerular Filtration rate	How well kidneys work Measures creatinine in blood	Same as above	Same as above

Name	Meaning	Descriptor/What it does	High	Low
AST (SGOT)	Aspartame Amino transferase, liver producing enzyme	Is one of the two liver enzymes viral hepatitis-liver function test	Yellow skin or eyes, jaundice, tiredness weakness, swollen belly stomach pain loss of appetite, itchy skin, dark colored urine, light colored poop, swelling in legs, ankle bruises, fatty liver disease	Pregnancy, good health, organs functioning properly
Sodium electrolyte	Source is salt controls heart pulse	Measures salt in blood	Frequent headaches heart attack, high blood pressure	Low electrolytes may cause high blood pressure
Potassium electrolyte	Source is food	Measures potassium in blood	Nausea, slow, weak, or irregular pulse	Muscular contraction weakness nervous system failures
Chloride electrolyte	Source is salt	Measures chloride in blood	Hyperchloremia chloride essential for body	Hypochloremia fluid loss, dehydration, vomiting weakness,high blood pH
CO2	Carbon dioxide	Measures CO2 in blood	Cushing Disease metabolic alkalosis	May indicate medical condition
CA C Calcium CT Scan		Heart scan to detect calcified plaque, fats, & cholesterol Measures C-reactive protein	Deposits in arteries increase risk of heart attack, need for statins, calcified plaque Increased level of inflammation	Malnutrition and low metabolism

Name	Meaning	Descriptor/What it does	High	Low
Albumin		Measures albumin in bloodstream Carries hormones, vitamins & enzymes in blood stream	Dehydration or high protein diet usually not serious	May indicate lives or kidney problems
Gamma globulin	Measures c-reactive protein	Measures levels of protein in blood	Increased inflammation	Weakened immunity multiple myeloma
A/G ratio	Albulim/Globulin	Measures ratio		When ratio is low, disease is developing
Billirubin		Yellow substance found in blood when red blood cells break down	Jaundice, liver disease, anemia yellowish eyes, gallstone illeus	Low Billirubin is of no concern for abnormalities
ALT (SGPT)	Alanine	Measures ALT in blood	Liver problem detected before liver	No disorder
	Amino Tranferase Pyruvic Transaminase	Liver enzyme	Disease develops	Yellow skin and eyes
ALP	Alkaline Phospatase	Measures ATP in blood stream	Diagnosis of hepatobiliary Sign of bone disorder and turnover	No disorder

Name	Meaning	Descriptor/What it does	High	Low
Uric Acid		Measures uric acid in bloodstream Normal waste product	Diagnose gout, rapid cell turnover for people undergoing chemotherapy or radiation treatment for cancer	No disorder
Iron		Measures iron in blood	Indicates iron toxicity	Anemia, iron deficiency
Ferritin iron		Measures iron stored inside cells	Potential dementia	
Serum iron		Measures iron stored inside body		
TIBC	Transferrin and iron Binding capacity	Measures iron in blood, Test ordered when hemoglobin reserve capacity of transferrin portion not yet saturated with iron, sideroblastic anemia (page 22)	Excess iron causes problems iron toxicity	Anemia, thalassemia (page 21) microcytes are small pale red blood cells, iron deficiency, hemolytic anemia, hemochromatosis (page 22)
UIBC	Unsaturated Iron-Binding Capacity	Evaluates iron deficiency or iron overload reserve capacity	Cirrhosis, scarring of liver, circulation limit by the heart, hemachromatosis, damage to pancreas leads to diabetes	UIBC test is used with a serum binding test and a TIBC test to evaluate people suspected of iron deficiency or overload

Name	Meaning	Descriptor/What it does	High	Low
Ferritin		Measures iron in blood iron deficiency	Microcytic: blood cells not yet hepalitis, developed inflammation, dehydration overactive protein prevents blood clotting	Anemia, tiredness, fatigue feet swelling, weakness fatigue liver disease, diziness, numbness
protein		Hypoproteinemia low =	Low level of protein	Overactive protein prevents blood clotting
C-reactive protein		An annular ring-shaped entamic protein found in blood plasma Binds to dead cells indicates overactive cytokines Indicates inflammation chronic disease infection	>3	<1

CHAPTER 2

Lipid Panel

		High	Low
Cholesterol	Measures amount of cholesterol Calculated: Total Cholesterol = LDL + HDL + 1/4 Triuglycerides	Deposits in arteries as fats HDL is good cholesterol, LDL & triglycerides are bad High LDL is an indication of developing heart disease, gallstones	Less is better
Triglycerides	Measures fats found in bloodstream	Indications of potential heart blockage	Less is better
HDL	Measure high density lipoproteins	Called: Good cholesterol -consumes LDL	Higher is better
LDL Cholesterol	Measure low density lipoproteins	Plaque build-up in arteries risk of heart disease	Less is better
Ratio:	Calculates; Cholesterol/HDL	Lower is better	Higher is not good

CHAPTER 3

Complete Blood Count

		High	**Low**
WBC White Blood Count	Measures white cells in blood	Predictive of death	bone marrow failure leukocyte count crowds out red blood cells autoimmune disorder serious bacterial infection mononucleosis
RBC Red Blood Cells Erythrocyte count	Measure of oxygen carried in blood	Undiagnosed illness fatigue	Red blood cells crowding Cells = leukemia
Leukocytes	White blood cells in urine	Infection is possible	Infection is unlikely anemia, polycythemia vera
Hemoglobin	Measures hemoglobin in blood Carries oxygen to organs and tissues Transports carbon dioxide back to lungs Hemoglobin is a protein inside red blood cells	Bone marrow not working	

		High	**Low**
Hematocrit Red blood cells	Measures how much of blood (erythrocytes) is red blood cells	Heart disease, dehydration, scarring or thickening of lungs, bone marrow disease Obstructive sleep apnea, smoking, COPD (chronic obstructive pulmonary disease) Increased blood viscosity, polyglobulia, - Hemocrit is a bit higher than normal	Anemia fatigue, headaches dizziness polycythemia **vera**
MCV Mean corpuscular volume	Measures average volume of a red blood cell used with red cell distribution width to assess anemia	Differentiate anemia from other causes	Low hemoglobin concentration microcytic anemia (small blood cell anemia) may need transfusion
MCH Mean corpuscular Hemoglobin	Measures amount of hemoglobin red blood cells can contain	Can be a sign of disease	Can be a sign of disease
MCHC Mean Corpuscular Hemoglobin Concentration	Hemoglobin/Red Blood Cell Count	Hyperchromia or macrocytic anemia	Anemia, fatigue, pale, general weakness

		High	Low
RDW Red Cell Distribution width	Measures size of red blood cells or volume of red blood cells use to diagnose blood disorders combined with other tests	High RDW and High MCV means anemia lack of folate or B-12-liver not functioning well High RDW and low MCV means anemia of body tests	Macrocycytic distribution distribution of red blood cells not enough to satisfy needs of body, means Blood cells are small and uniforms in size, testing error
Platelets	Platelets (thrombocytes) in the Blood measures average number of platelets	Thrombocytosis, anemia, iron deficiency, usually not a problem	Thrombocytopenia poor clotting stops bleeding by forming plugs in bone marrow
MPV Mean Platelet volume	Measures average size of platelets	Thrombocythemia-may require low dose such as ecotrin or heparin to thin the blood headaches, dizziness, light headedness are symptoms	Microcytic, macrocytic normocytic

CHAPTER 4

White Blood Cells

		High	Low
Netrophils	Type of white blood cell 55-70% of total white blood cell count In bone marrow	Neutrophilic leukocytosis Seldom poses risk of infections usually asymptomatic, Pregnancy stress, bacterial infections underlying medical conditions	Neutropenia-vulnerable to infections
Lymphocytes	Measures B & T lymphocytes & killer Protects cells from bacterial and viral infections	Bacterial infection viral infection, cancer of the blood or lymphatic system, lymphatic system, autoimmune disorder that causes chronic inflammation, low count is called lymphocytopenia	Lymphoctyopenia AIDS, typhoid fever caused by salmonella viral hepatitis when liver becomes injured or infected

		High	Low
Monocytes	Largest white blood cell-circulate in blood to become macrophages or dendritic cells that Protect agaist viral, bacterial, fungal & Protozoa infections & cancer	Higher is better	Bacterial and viral infections inflamed and stiff joints
Eosinophils	White blood cell that destroys invading germs, responds to inflammation and slows progression of kidney disease	Hypereosinophilia eosinophils do their job and go away	Eosinopenia, drunkiness near zero is normal range asthmatic patients Cushing Syndrom, blood Stream infection, (sepsis) Low usually not a problem
Basophils 0.5-1% of White blood cells	White blood cells, changes can indicate if patient suffering from illness, autoimmune disease, created in response to types of leukemia, inflamation and infection-responsible for phagocytosis immune cells eating other cells	Basophilia indicates hives, inflammation, ood allergies, Crohn's disease, certain types of leukemia, conditions causing too many white blood cells are produced	Acute infection, cancer, severe injury, severe allergies, women under stress, hyperthyoidism (over active throid)
Immature Granulocytes	Measures immature white blood cells healthy people do not show these cells Measures hemoglobin in blood	Means that body is fighting an infection to the bone marrow, cancerous diseases or pregnancy, may include metamyelocytes, myelocytes, & promyelocytes	Granulocytosis, reduce body's ability to fight infections, anemia, leukemia

		High	**Low**
Neutrophils Absolute	Neutrophils are one of five types of cells leucocytes assessment of neutrophils that fight infection in bloodstream	Active bacterial infection, rarely from cancer or leukemia, sometimes from stress	Diseases & treatments, and are result of cancer thermography and neutropenia
Lymphocytes Absolute	White blood cells that include-cells, T-cells, & natural killer cells	HIV-AIDS, bone marrow failure chemotherapy viral infections, leukemia, lymphoma, monocytes	bacterial infection, viral infection, cancer of the blood or Lymphatic System autoimmune disorder causing inflammation
Monocytes Absolute	Largest type of white blood cell accompanied by low red blood cells	higher is better	Oxygen content low, Protects body from pathogens in gastrointestinal tract, and urinary tract, cause could be vitamin deficiency, anemia or stress, wipe out blood cells faster than body can make them
Eosinophils Absolute	Measure one type of blood cell destroys invading germs and creates inflammatory response produced in bone marrow	Becomes active during certain allergic diseases & infections, parasites, or asthma, adrenal condition toxins, autoimmune disease endocrine disorders certain medications	usually not a problem alcohol intoxication, bone marrow disorder production of steroids such as corticosal low (eosinopenia)

		High	Low
Basophils absolute	Largest type of mature white blood cell	severe allergies,under sudden emotional or physical l stress called basophilia indicating hives, inflammation, Crohn's disease basophenia (low count) Absolute Food allergies, leukemia	low count uncommon allergic reaction or hyperthyroidism
Immature granulocyte absolute	type of white blood cell that leaves bone a bit early before maturity	due to many philological conditions, usually an active bacterial infection in the body	low number of certain white blood cells neutrophils that increases susceptibility to infection more, Frequent infections
NRBC%	Number of nucleated Red blood cells in a sample of blood-normally found in the circulation of a fetus	associated with increased mortality	infection, inflammation, dietary deficiency causing anemia . hemoglobin variants such as sickle cell anemia shortness of breath, and fatigue
Hemoglobin A1c	Measures the concentration of glucose (sugar) in blood stream that is attached to hemoglobin (protean in blood that Carries oxygen	type 2 diabetes or risk of developing diabetes	lower is better

		High	Low
TSH Throid Stimulating Hormone	Measures the thyroid hormone Measures the amount of TSH in the blood Regulates how body uses energy also Regulates weight, body temperature, Muscle strength, & mood	potential thyroid disorder, hyperthyroidism Grave's disease an autoimmune disorder	potential thyroid disorder hypothyroidism, thyroid gland disease
Glucose C2H1206	Blood sugar main energy source Makes cellulose for cell walls	Diabetes but other high sugar Foods and or medicines	Hyperglycemia excessive blood Poor wound healing, weight loss Leave no space for lower sentences
Lead	drinking water	decreased Vitamin A, anemia, acute central nervous Disorder	no disadvantage
Mercury	tuna and large fish	damage to nervous system especially the brain nervousness, anxiety, irritability, depression, memory loss	no disadvantage

		High	Low
Immuno-globulin also known as anitibodies	immune globulins are proteins made by the immune system to fight diseases causing substances like viruses and bacteria, Five tests iGA, igD, igE, igD, and igM positive results indicate natural immunity	allergies, overactive immune system, multiple myeloma long term hepatitis, multiple sclerosis, in the blood stream leukemia. auto-immune disease, cancer	igG is the most antibody There are 4 igGs I gG1, igG2, igG3, & igG4 Iif these are low then immune system is not working properly low igG can also be caused by steroids Low igG and iGa caused infection and auto-immunity disease

CHAPTER 5

Thyroid

		High	Low
Thyroxine Total (T4)	Measures the amount of the T4 hormone in the blood T4 is produced by the throid gland, The hypothalamus and pituitary glands control the release of T4. There is a total T4 that measures the amount of thyroxine circulating in the blood. A Free T4 measures what is not bound and able to freely enter and effect body tissues	can indicate disease, hyperthyroidism Total T4 levels are affected by medication	can indicate disease hypothyroidism T4 are affected by levels are affected by medication
T3 Uptake	Measures the amount of thyroid related Binding proteins that are in the blood This includes albumin and TBG (Thyroid Binding Protein)	more TBG is bound to T4 or T3 may indicate abnormalities, low T3 may indicate starvation hyperthyroidism	testing is not always helpful

CHAPTER 6

Vitamins

		High	Low
Vitamin B12 Folate	Measures folate in blood stream B-12 Called cobalamin, affects methylation it is the transfer of four atoms - one carbon atom and 3 hydrogen atoms (CH3 When from one substance goes to another. optimal) methylation occurs, it has a significant positive impact on many biochemical reactions in the body that regulate the activity of the neurological, reproductive, and detoxification systems, including those relating to methylation which is a simple biochemical process	headaches, irritability, insomnia, running nose, body pain, itchy skin	diagnose macrocytic anemia malnutrition or malabsorbtion fatigue, insomnia, , depression) addiction obsessive compulsive, disorder delusions, allergies headaches, digestive cardiovascular concerns, low tolerance for pain, high libido lack of motivatioin missing and component of immunological recovery

Vitamin E	Measures vitamin E in blood Foods with Vitamin E; sunflower seeds, Kiwi, spinach, blackberries,mangoes, Resberries, nectarines, blueberries, apricots, Plumbs, grapes, rhubarb, oranges, apples cantelope, olives, grapefruit, almonds strawberries	muscle weakness, central nervous system Problems, coordination and walking difficulties Purkinje neurons break, numbness Purkinje cells, also called Purkinje neurons, are neurons in vertebrate animals located in the cerebellar cortex of the brain Purkinje cell bodies are shaped like a flask and have many threadlike extensions called dendrites, which receive impulses from other neurons called granule cells	bleeding, slow clotting
Vitamin B-12	B-12 Measures how much B-12 is in the blood stream B-12 makes red blood cells that transport oxygen affects methylation B1 called Thiamine, B2 is riboflavin B3 is nicotinic acid niacin B5 pantothenic acid, B6 is pyridoxine Foods rich in Vitamin B fortified cereals, salmon, tuna, cod, haddock, fortified soy milk Greek plain non-fat yogurt, swiss cheese eggs beans, bananas, lentils, peppers	fatigue, nervousness, dizziness, numbness tingling in fingers and toes, long term; loss of mobility, problems walking, memory loss, nerve damage accompanied by low, red blood 200 - 400 milligrams/L is recommended by Dr. Micozzi ageing may be a result of Vit B deficiency essential to produce serotonin, melatonin, & dopamine, & healthy nerves	malnutrition of B-12 weakness, tingling, numbness Electric shock feelings for no reason pyridoxine balance, mental confusion, forgetfullness anemia, Yellow tinge to skin anemia, swollen red tongue, ulcers pins and needles sparaesthesia Grave's Disease chronoic fatigue, trembling memory disorder, muscle weakness, difficult to concentrate, tremors, tinnitus shortness of breath, anemia low absorbtion of iron

Vitamin D	Vitamin D controls calcium and phosphate levels in the body 50 – 75 micromol/L is recommended Dr. Icozzi	nausea, vomiting, calcium buildup in blood weakness frequent urination, progression to bone pain, kidney problems such as calcium stones, weight Loss in short time	bone metabolism, 1, 25 parathyroid function hypocalcemia, renal osteodystrophy or chronic renal failure , bone density, Skeletal fractures, risk of falling
Vitamin A	Measures VitaminA in bloodstream Foods with Vitamin A. mango, watermelon Liver, lamb, cod liver oil, cantaloupe, grapefruit, Apricot, nectarines, carrots, squash, cheese, Promotes: eye health,healthy teeth and skin	Hypervitaminosis, drowsiness, irritability, Abdominal pain, nausea, increased pressure on the Brain, diarrhea, joint pain, bone pain, birth defects, Liver damage, increased calcium in blood, rash, Dizziness, headaches	swelling of bones, dry skin, mouth ulcer, confusion & vision changes
Vitamin C	Measure Vitamin C in bloodstream acid foods rich in Vitamin C strawberries, broccoli, potatoes acerola black cherries, potatoes peas, papaya peppers kale, cantaloupe makes collagen, strengthens skin protects skin elasticity, supports weight loss	diarrhea, vomiting, heartburn, abdominal cramps headaches, insomnia, gastrointestinal disturbance cramping, bloating, kidney stones, birth defects, swelling, weakened bones, poor immune function	rough bumpy skin, called ascorbic keratosis pilaris, peppers, corkscrew body hairs scurvy, faigue, impaired wound't, healing, chronic pain, rough skin, shortened breath depression, bleeding, anemia, irregular heartbeat, feet & muscle Tissue becomes weakness, unsteady confusion, forgetfulness, bruising gum tissue movement gum Loss, numbness or tingling inhands, weak and heals slowly Low energy, bad moods

Prostate	Foods that minimize prostate growth Siurce: Dr. marc Micolli, PhD	tomatoes, blueberries, broccoli, legumes, fatty fish	

The following foods are associated with longevity: dark chocolate, garlic, cinnamon, olive oil, & honey. These contain essential nutrients. **Olive oil** contains polyphenols that slows down cardiovascular and neurodegenerative diseases and cancer and a lower risk of osteoporosis **Dark Chocolate** are rich in flavanols that protect the heart. **Cinnamon** reduces body inflammation root cause of most chronic diseases. **Garlic** Increases production of lymphocytes & macrophages that attack foreign bodies. Allicin is a sulfur compound that prevents certain cancers and helps to lower blood sugar cholesterol & blood pressure and protects against infecttions **Pure or raw honey** has vitamins C, K, E, B-2, B-3, B-5 & B-6

Vitamin K Test	Measures Vitamin K in the bloodstream asparagus, fresh dry basil, soybeans, cucumbers, extra virgin olive oil, kale, leafy greens, brussels sprouts, broccoli, prunes, scallions, cabbage	low potential for toxicityside effects from medication decreased appetite, enlarged liver, swelling, muscle coordination Stiffness, fast and/or weak heartbeat yellow eyes or skin paleness	bleeding from marea of cut umbilicil bleeding on skin & easily bruising, heavy high billirubin, premature babies, itching and heavy periods, risk of bone fracture, side redness, upset stomach effects So far, research shows vitamin K helps to prevent calcification (and hardening) of soft tissues such as blood vessels that need to remain elastic and flexible. We also know vitamin K has an important role in the formation of healthy bones. third, we know vitamin K helps with the function of insulin to lower blood sugar and nourish the cells with needed calories.

Sed Rate (ESR)	Erythrocyte Sedimentation Rate measures the rate the red blood cells separate from a sample of blood that has been treated to prevent clotting Erythrocytes are red blood cells. The test reveals Inflammatory activity in the body arising from autoimmune disease, infections, or tumors	Indicates more inflammation	Indicates less inflammation
Carbon Dioxide	This measures the CO2 in the blood stream much or too little maybe electrolyte imbalance weakness, fatigue, prolonged vomiting diarrhea	lung disease, Cushing Syndrome (make too much cortisol) adrenal gland disorder hormonal disorders, alkalosis (too much base in the blood) – high Ph)	Addison's disease, dizziness weight loss, dehydration, acidosis (too much acid in the blood complication of type 1 and type 2 diabetes
Coffee	Source: MNarc Micozzi, MD, PhD	lowers risk of skin cancer, colin cancer, cardio-Vascular disease, brain disease	
Cayenne source:	MNarc Micozzi, MD, PhD contains capsaicin, source of Vitamins C, A, B-8, & K	lowers blood pressure, promotes digestive health, Lowers pain when applied to skin, improves vein Strength, forestalls blood clots, protects against Alzheimer's, Parkinson's, & type II diabetes	
Iron		builds muscles and maintains Healthy blood Zinc helps wounds heal, makes Proteins and DNA, healthy immune system	

CHAPTER 7

Definitions

Immunocompromised
neutrophils made in bone marrow Neutropils travel throughout the body, sense infections Gather at the infection destroy the pathogen deficient number of white blood cells, deficient antibodies

need adequate supply and size of white blood cells

invasion by bacteria, fungi, viruses, and other pathogens that cause infections, anemia if too few blood cells to carry O2

BMI			
BMI	Body Mass Index	Patient considers overweight if BMI > 30	lower is healthier <30
	Weight (kilograms)/Height^2 (meters)	Patient considers overweight if BMI > 30	lower is healthier <30
	Weight (lbs)/Height^2 (inches^2) X 700		

PSA Prostate Specific Antigen Might indicate large prostate but cannot be interpreted lower is better as evidence of the presence or absence of a malignancy. An antigen any substance (such as an immunogenic or a hapten) foreign to the body that evokes an immune response either alone or after forming a complex with a larger molecule (such as a protein) and that is capable of binding with a product (such as an antibody or T cell) of the immune response. (Haptens are small molecules that elicit an immune response only when attached to a large carrier such as a protein; the carrier may be one that also does not elicit an immune response by itself- in general only large molecules, infectious agents or insoluble foreign matter can elicit an immune response in the body.) This means your immune system does not recognize the substance, and is trying to fight it Off. An antigen may be a substance from the environment, such as chemicals, bacteria, viruses, or pollen. An antibody (Ab), also known as an immunoglobulin (Ig), is a large, Y-shaped protein used by the immune system to identify and neutralize foreign objects such as pathogenic bacteria and viruses. The antibody recognizes a unique molecule of the pathogen, called an antigen. Each tip of the "Y" of an antibody contains a paratope (analogous to a lock) that is specific for one particular epitope (the part of an antigen that is recognized by the antibody).

Antigen | Definition of Antigen by Merriam-Webster
Antigen definition is - any substance (such as an immunogen or a hapten) foreign to the body that evokes an immune response either alone or after forming a complex with a larger molecule (such as a protein) and that is capable of binding with a product (such as an antibody or T cell) of the immune response. An antigen is any substance that causes your immune system to produce antibodies against it. This means your immune system does not recognize the substance, and is trying to fight it off. An antigen may be a substance from the environment, such as chemicals, bacteria, viruses, or pollen. An antigen may also form inside the body

Alkalosis | Definition of alkalosis by Medical dictionary
alkalosis. (ăl'kə-lō'sĭs) n. 1. Abnormally high alkalinity of the blood and body tissues caused by an excess of bicarbonates, as from an increase in alkali intake, or by or a deficiency of acids other than carbonic acid, as from vomiting also called metabolic alkalosis. Alkalosis occurs when your body has too many bases (high Ph). It can occur due to decreased blood levels of carbon dioxide, which is an acid. It can also occur due to increased blood levels of bicarbonate.

Alkalosis is a condition of the blood and other body fluids in which the bicarbonate concentration is above normal, tending toward alkalemia. What does alkalosis mean? It means an abnormally high alkalinity of the blood and body fluids. Alkalosis is the result of a process reducing hydrogen ion concentration of arterial blood plasma. In contrast to acidemia, alkalemia occurs when the serum pH is higher than normal. Alkalosis is usually divided into the categories of respiratory alkalosis and metabolic alkalosis or a combined respiratory/metabolic alkalosis. Metabolic alkalosis is a pH imbalance in which the body has accumulated too much of an alkaline substance, such as bicarbonate, and does not have enough acid to effectively neutralize the effects of the alkalinity.

Antibody | Definition of Antibody by Merriam-Webster
Antibody definition is - any of a large number of proteins of high molecular weight that are produced normally by specialized B cells after stimulation by an antigen and act specifically against the antigen in an immune response, that are produced abnormally by some cancer cells, and that typically consist of four subunits including two heavy chains and two light chains —called also immunoglobulin.

An antibody is a protein component of the immune system that circulates in the blood, recognizes foreign substances like bacteria and viruses, and neutralizes them. After exposure to a foreign substance, called an antigen, antibodies continue to circulate in the blood, providing protection against future exposuses to that antigen.

Monoclonal antibody
A monoclonal antibody (mAb or moAb) is an antibody made by cloning a unique white blood cell. All subsequent antibodies derived this way trace back to a unique parent cell Monoclonal antibodies can have monovalent affinity binding only to the same epitope (the part of an antigen that is recognized by the antibody). In contrast, polyclonal antibodies bind to multiple epitopes and are usually made by several different antibody secreting plasma cell lineages. Specific monoclonal antibodies can also be engineered, by increasing the therapeutic targets of one monoclonal antibody to two epitopes. It is possible to produce monoclonal antibodies that specifically bind to virtually any suitable substance; they can then serve to detect or purify it. This capability has become an important tool in biochemistry, molecular biology, and medicine.

Folate (Cambridge Dictionary)
A type of B vitamin essential for cell growth and reproduction. It is found in leafy green leaves, legumes, liver, eggs, and fresh fruits.

Cytokines
Cytokines are soluble proteins that act as chemical messengers in the immune response, and play an important role for communication with cells in other systems and in cell growth, differentiation, and hematopoisis. New advances have shown that there may be wide implications for cytokines in the diagnosis and treatment of various disorders. Cytokines have been implicated in cancer, autoimmune disorders, and septic shock, among other disorders. The basal concentration of circulating cytokines is very low and usually in range of only a few picograms per milliliter.

Hematopoisis occurs in the marrow of the long bones such as the femur and tibia. In adults, it occurs mainly in the pelvis, cranium, vertebrae, and sternum and In some cases, the liver, thymus, and spleen may resume their haematopoietic function, if necessary. This is called extramedullary haematopoisis.

Thalassemia is an inherited (i.e., passed from parents to children through genes) blood disorder caused when the body does not make enough of a protein called hemoglobin, an important part of red blood cells.

Hemochromatosis is a hereditary disease that causes your body to absorb too much iron from the food you eat. Excess iron is stored in your organs, especially your liver, heart and pancreas. iron from the food you eat. Excess iron is stored in your organs, especially your liver, heart and pancreas. Too much iron can lead to life-threatening conditions, such as liver disease, heart problems and diabetes.

Aplastic anemia where the bone marrow produces ringed sideroblasts rather than healthy red blood cells (erythrocytes) Sideroblastic anemia, or sideroachrestic anemia, is a form of anemia in which the bone marrow produces ringed sideroblasts rather than healthy red blood cells (erythrocytes). In sideroblastic anemia, the body has iron available but cannot incorporate it into hemoglobin, which red blood cells need in order to transport oxygen efficiently.

Cortisol is most commonly known as the body's stress hormone. It is a hormone that regulates stress, metabolism, the "fight-or-flight" response, and many other important functions. It's made by the adrenal glands. Levels and usage are regulated by the hypothalamus, pituitary, and adrenals (HPA axis).: Your body functions best when cortisol is at optimal levels. "Cortisol is a steroid hormone that your own body makes," explains Disha Narang, MD, an endocrinologist from Chicago and a member of Endocrine Web's Editorial Board. "If someone has a bad backache or infection, doctors will administer steroids to decrease inflammation. Cortisol is your body's own way of doing that internally." It is produced from cholesterol molecules within the adrenal glands (the zona fasciculata layer to be exact) and regulated by the hypothalamic-pituitary-adrenal glands . In simpler terms, cortisol is produced in the kidneys There are 300 empirical articles describing a relationship between psychological stress and the immune system parameters (immunoglobulin).

New studies claim that babies that are left alone to cry repeatedly develop elevated of the stress hormone cortisol in their blood. Numerous studies suggest that high cortisol levels are toxic to a newborn's developing brain. This has a profound negative effect on physical and mental health as well as a disruption in their metabolism and digestion. This also leads to increased blood pressure and risk of plaque build-up. High levels of cortisol narrow down the arteries which lead to increased blood pressure. Untended babies may have a profound effect in their later life. Cortisol can be measured by a blood test.

CHAPTER 8

Other Tests

CareStart Covid-19 (swab nose mucus) by Access Bio	Antigen Reagent manufactured for short test (results in 20 minutes)	If mucus added to the reagent turns blue, Covid-19 is present Long test swabs deeper in nose for long test (3 days)	no blue means Covid -19 is absent
Urine test indication	Urine compose of carbon oxygen, hydrogen, & nitrogen (COHN) + chloride, sodium potassium & creatinine	dark amber color or other colors may depend on diet beets turn urine red, (blood can also turn urine red), colored beverages may turn urine green or from a urinary tract infection	no color or low color not an illness

Does Rebounding Exercise Increase White Blood Cell Count?

Exercise causes change in antibodies and white blood cells (WBC). WBCs are the body's immune system cells that fight disease. WBCs are the body's immune system cells that fight disease. These antibodies or WBCs circulate more rapidly, so they could detect illnesses earlier than they might have before. Exercise naturally causes increased white blood cell production. In fact, your white blood cell count could increase threefold after a moderate workout session and remain at that level for an hour or more after finishing your workout. A higher white blood cell count improves your resistance to infections and illness. Potential exercise options include brisk walking, bicycling and participation in relatively slow-paced games like golf. Typically, the intensity and duration of exercise required to boost your white blood cells are less than those required by a rigorous aerobic exercise routine, White and red blood cells are made in bone marrow. Stress and immunity.

CHAPTER 9

Other Diseases

Crohn's disease - Symptoms
is a type of inflammatory bowel disease (IBD) that may affect any segment of the gastrointestinal tract from the mouth to the anus. Symptoms often include abdominal pain, diarrhea (which may be bloody if inflammation is severe), fever, abdominal distension, and weight loss. Other complications outside the gastrointestinal tract may include anemia, skin rashes, arthritis, and inflammation.

Graves' disease - Symptoms and causes - Mayo Clinic
Graves' disease is an immune system disorder that results in the overproduction of thyroid hormones (hyperthyroidism). Although a number Of disorders may result in hyperthyroidism. Graves' disease is a common cause. Thyroid hormones affect many body systems, so signs of symptoms of Graves 'disease can be wide ranging. The symptoms of Graves' disease include: weight loss despite increased appetite. faster heart rate, higher blood pressure, increased nervousness, excessive perspiration and increased sensitivity. Graves' disease is an autoimmune disorder that causes hyperthyroidism, or overactive thyroid. With this disease, your immune system attacks the thyroid and causes it to make more thyroid hormone than your body needs. The thyroid is a small, butterfly-shaped gland in the front of your neck. Graves' disease is an autoimmune disease that affects the thyroid gland. The gland produces too much thyroid hormone, a condition known as hyperthyroidism. Thyroid hormones regulate body temperature, heart rate and metabolism.

An overactive thyroid causes problems with organs like the heart, as well as bones and muscles. Graves' disease is the most commoncause of hyperthyroidism, so some Graves' disease symptoms are the same as hyperthyroidism symptoms. However, people with Graves' disease may also have other symptoms not related to hyperthyroidism. It can be a challenge to detect Graves' disease early on. Graves' eye disease can cause dry and red irritated eyes, bulging eyes, and shortened eyelids that won't close all the way. Your symptoms may stay stable for a while or get better or worse.

Polycythemia vera - Symptoms and causes - Mayo Clinic
Polycythemia vera (pol-e-sy-THEE-me-uh VEER-uh) is a type of blood cancer. It causes your bone marrow to make too many red blood cells. These excess cells thicken your blood, slowing its flow, which may cause serious problems, such as blood clots. Polycythemia vera is rare. Polycythemia vera is a condition characterized by an increased number of red blood cells in the bloodstream (erythrocytosis). Affected people may also have excess white blood cells and platelets. Conditions where the body makes too many of these cells are known as myeloproliferative neoplasms. The increase in blood cells makes the blood thicker. Thick blood can lead to strokes or tissue and organ damage

Thalassemia - Symptoms and causes - Mayo Clinic
There are several types of thalassemia. The signs and symptoms you have depend on the type and severity of your condition. Thalassemia signs and symptoms can include: fatigue; weakness; pale or yellowish skin; facial bone deformities; slow growth; abdominal swelling; dark urine. Alpha thalassemia silent carriers generally have no signs or symptoms of the disorder. People who have alpha or beta thalassemia trait can have mild anemia.

When there are not enough healthy red blood cells, there is also not enough oxygen delivered to all the other cells of the body, which may cause a person to feel tired, weak or short of breath. This is a condition called anemia. People with thalassemia may have mild or severe anemia.People who have hemoglobin disease or beta thalassemia major (also called Cooley's anemia) have severe thalassemia. Signs and symptoms usually occur within the first 2 years of life. They may include severe anemia and other health problems, such as: A pale and listless appearance; Poor appetite. There are two main types of thalassemia, alpha thalassemia and beta thalassemia. Signs and symptoms vary but may include mild to severe anemia, paleness, fatigue, yellow discoloration of skin (jaundice), and bone problems. People who have thalassemia produce fewer healthy hemoglobin proteins, and their bone marrow produces fewer healthy red blood cells. Thalassemias can cause mild or severe anemia and other complications that can occur over time (such as iron overload). Symptoms of anemia include fatigue, difficulty breathing, dizziness, and a pale skin tone. Thalassemia is an inherited blood condition. If you have it, your body has fewer red blood cells and less hemoglobin than it should. Hemoglobin is important because it lets your red blood cell provide the brain with oxygen.

Thrombocytosis - Symptoms and causes - Mayo Clinic
Thrombocytosis (throm-boe-sie-TOE-sis) is a disorder in which your body produces too many platelets. It's called reactive thrombocytosis or secondary thrombocytosis when the cause is an underlying condition, such as an infection. Less commonly, when thrombocytosis has no apparent underlying condition as a cause, the disorder is called primary thrombocythemia or essential thrombocythemia.

Thrombocytosis is an abnormally increased number of platelets in the blood. Platelets are blood cells that stick together, helping blood to clot. Thrombocytosis is a condition that may have many causes.

Throbocytosis is classified as one of two types. Platelets are blood cells in plasma that stop bleeding by sticking together to form a clot. Too many platelets can lead to certain conditions, such as stroke, heart attack or a clot in the blood vessels. Medical Definition of thrombocytosis : increase and especially abnormal increase in the number of platelets in the blood that typically occurs in association with a myeloproliferative disorder (as thrombocythemia or chronic myelogenous leukemia) or as a nonspecific response to an underlying disorder or disease (as a systemic infection) also called thrombocythemia.

Thrombocythemia (THROM-bo-si-THE-me-ah) and thrombocytosis (THROM-bo-si-TO-sis) are conditions in which your blood has a higher than normal number of platelets (PLATE-lets). Platelets are blood cell fragments. They're made in your bone marrow along with other kinds of blood cells. There are two types: essential thrombocythemia and reactive thrombocytosis. Essential thrombocythemia arises on its own, whereas reactive thrombocytosis is caused by another ondition. Thrombocytosis is defined as a platelet count above 450,000/ μL, which is typically considered the upper limit of the normal laboratory reference range of 150,000 to 450,000/μL. Thrombocytosis is very frequently detected as an incidental laboratory abnormality and subsequently a causal explanation is sought

Addison's Disease - Symptoms and causes

Addison's disease, also known as primary adrenal insufficiency, is a rare long-term endocrine disorder characterized by inadequate production of the steroid hormones cortisol and aldosterone by the two outer layers of the cells of the adrenal glands (adrenal cortex). Addison's disease Damage to the adrenal glands in Addison's disease is usually caused by autoimmune disease—when your immune system attacks your body's own cells and organs. In developed countries, autoimmune disease causes 8 or 9 of every 10 cases of Addison's disease. Certain infections can also cause Addison's disease. Adrenal insufficiency occurs when the adrenal glands don't make enough of the hormone cortisol. The primary kind is known as Addison's disease. Addison's disease, or hypoadrenocorticism, is caused by a lower-than-normal production of hormones, like cortisol, by the adrenal glands, which are small glands located near the kidneys. Adrenal hormones are necessary to control salt, sugar, and water balance in the body.

Cushings syndrome vs. Cushings disease - MedicineNet

What is the difference between Cushing's syndrome and Cushing's disease? Any condition that causes the adrenal gland to produce excessive cortisol results in the disorder Cushing's syndrome. Cushing syndrome is characterized by facial and torso obesity, high blood pressure, stretch marks on the belly, weakness, osteoporosis, and facial hair growth in females. Cushing's disease is not the same as Cushing's syndrome. Cushing's syndrome refers to the general state characterized by excessive levels of cortisol in the blood. Elevated cortisol levels can occur for reasons other than a pituitary tumor, including: tumors of the adrenal glands producing cortisol, Cushing disease and Cushing syndrome are two endocrine conditions which take place due to over production of a-fore mentioned Cortisol. Cushing disease is caused by a tumor or an excessive growth in the pituitary gland and the disease is a major cause of the Cushing syndrome. This is the main difference between Cushing disease and Cushing syndrome

Multiple myeloma (MM) Symptoms and causes
also known as plasma cell myeloma and simply myeloma, is a cancer of plasma cells, a type of white blood cell that normally produces antibodies. Often, no symptoms are noticed initially. As it progresses, bone pain, anemia, kidney dysfunction, and infections may occur. Complications may include amyloidosis

Hepatobiliary Medical Definition | Merriam-Webster Medical ...
Hepatobiliary relates to the liver and bile, bile ducts, and gallbladder . For example, MRI (magnetic resonance imaging) can be applied to the hepatobiliary system. Hepatobiliary makes sense since "hepato-" refers to the liver and "-biliary" refers to the gallbladder, bile ducts, or bile. Hepatobiliary makes sense since "hepato-" refers to the liver and "biliary" refers to the gallbladder, or bile ducts. Inflammatory hepatobiliary disease is a generic term that comprises conditions presenting a complex noninfectious etiopathogenesis characterized by chronic inflammatory infiltrate and autoimmune features. Among these, the main distinction is based on the target tissue, whether this is the hepatocyte (as in the case of autoimmune hepatitis (AIH) or the bile duct cell (intrahepatic) small and medium sized in the case of primary biliary cirrhosis (PBC) or any level.

Hereditary hemochromatosis (he-moe-kroe-muh-TOE-sis)causes your body to absorb too much iron from the food you eat. Excess iron is stored in your organs, especially your liver, heart and pancreas. Too much iron. Hereditary hemochromatosis (he-moe-kroe-muh-TOE-sis) causes your body to absorb too much iron from the food you eat. Excess iron is stored in your organs, especially your liver, heart and pancreas. Too much iron can lead to life-threatening conditions, such as liver disease, heart problems, and diabetes.

Thrombocytosis - Symptoms and causes - Mayo Clinic
Thrombocytosis (throm-boe-sie-TOE-sis) is a disorder in which your body produces too many platelets. It's called reactive thrombocytosis or secondary thrombocytosis when the cause is an underlying condition, such as an infection. They're made in your bone marrow along with other kinds of blood cells.Thrombocytosis is an abnormally increased number of platelets in the blood. Platelets are blood cells that stick together, helping blood to clot. Thrombocytosis is a condition that may have many causes. Platelets are blood cell fragments. Throbocytosis is classified as one of two types.. Platelets are blood cells in plasma that stop bleeding by sticking together to form a clot.

Too many platelets can lead to certain conditions, including stroke, heart attack or a clot in the blood vessels. There are two types of thrombocytosis: primary and secondary. Thrombocytosis is a blood disorder that is marked by headaches, chest pain and loss of consciousness and can even be life-threatening for some sufferers. Thrombocythemia (THROM-bo-si-THE-me-ah) and thrombocytosis (THROM-bo-si-TO-sis) are conditions in which your blood has a higher than normal number of platelets (PLATE-lets).

Normocytic anemia

is a type of anemia and is a common issue that occurs for men and women typically over 85 years old. Its prevalence increases with age, reaching 44 percent in men older than 85 years. The most common type of normocytic anemia is anemia of chronic disease. Common symptoms include: fatigue dizziness or lightheadedness, dyspnea, exercise intolerance, generalized weakness, palpitation,headaches and decreased concentration.The issue is thought of as representing any of the following: an acute loss of blood of a substantial volume; a decreased production of normal-sized red blood cells (e.g., anemia of chronic disease, aplastic anemia); an increased production of HbS (Hemoglobulin Sickle) as seen in sickle cell (not sickle cell anemia). Chronic disease is the most common normocytic anemia and the second most common form of anemia worldwide after iron deficiency anemia.

The MCV (Mean Corpuscular Volume) may be low in some patients with this type of anemia The pathogenesis of anemia of chronic . disease is multifactorial and is related to hypoactivity of the bone marrow with relatively inadequate production of erythropoietin or a poor response to erytherythropoietin, as well as slightly shortened red blood cell survival.

Normocytic anemia characterized by proportionate decrease in hemoglobin, packed red cell volume, and number of erythrocytes per cubic millimeter of blood. Nutritional anemia anemia is due to a deficiency of an essential substance in the diet, which may be caused by poor dietary intake or by malabsorption; called also deficiency anemia. Normocytic anemia has many causes, the most common being anemia due to sudden blood loss, long-term diseases (chronic diseases), kidney failure, aplastic anemia, man-made heart valves or drug therapy. Anemia is a condition where there is a low level of a substance called hemoglobin in the blood. Normocytic normochromic anemia is one of the most common forms of anemia which is usually found along with other chronic diseases. A mild normocytic ormochromic anemia is a common occurrence found as a consequence of other diseases such as anemia due to chronic disorders or other disorders which include renal failure and acute blood loss.

Cortisol What causes low levels of cortisol?

Having lower-than-normal cortisol levels (hypocortisolism) is considered adrenal insufficiency. There are two types of adrenal insufficiency: primary and secondary. The causes of adrenal insufficiency include:

- **Primary adrenal insufficiency**: Primary adrenal insufficiency is most commonly caused by an autoimmune reaction in which your immune system attacks healthy cells in your adrenal glands for no known reason. This is called Addison's disease. Your adrenal glands can also become damaged from an infection or blood loss to the tissues (adrenal hemorrhage). All of these situations limit cortisol production.
- **Secondary adrenal insufficiency**: If you have an underactive pituitary gland (hypopituitarism) or a pituitary tumor, it can limit ACTH production. ACTH signals your adrenal glands to make cortisol, so limited ACTH results in limited cortisol production.

You can also have lower-than-normal cortisol levels after stopping treatment with corticosteroid medications, especially if you stop taking them very quickly after a long period of use.

What are the symptoms of low cortisol levels?

Symptoms of lower-than-normal cortisol levels, or adrenal insufficiency, include:

- Fatigue.
- Unintentional weight loss.
- Poor appetite.
- Low blood pressure (hypotension).
- Depression
- Heart Disease
- Immune System problems
- Obesity
- Chronic stress: cortisol levels become elevated and that leads to inflammation

Stress and Isolation Can Also Affect Your Physical Health

Mental health conditions often elicit a physiological response. Research suggests that people who feel more politically different than the average voters in their state experience more days of poor physical health each month. Fearing people with opposing viewpoints causes a constant state of "arousal and anxiety," Stress causes the brain to release the chemical cortisol, which regulates your body's response to stress. Dr. Michael Roeske (Psy D) of Mayo Clinic says moderate stress can actually be good for you, especially if you're "impassioned by it" and it's not preoccupying. Too much cortisol long-term can impact the immune system, and cause muscle weakness, high blood pressure, high blood sugar, and obesity. Chronic stress can make you irritable and cause conditions, like heart attacks, strokes, and chronic pain.

"We're not set up for this constant onslaught of stress around the political divisiveness that's happening now," Roeske says

CHAPTER 10

Idiopathic disease - Wikipedia

An idiopathic disease is any disease with an unknown cause or mechanism of apparent spontaneous origin. From Greek ἴδιος idios "one's own" and πάθος pathos "suffering", idiopathy means approximately "a disease of its own kind". For some medical conditions, one or more causes are somewhat understood, but in a certain percentage of people with the condition, the cause may not be readily apparent which has no known cause. For some medical conditions, one or more causes are somewhat understood, but in a certain percentage of cases Idiopathic is a medical term which is used to describe a condition. When a patient's case is described s idiopathic, it means that the doctor does not know what caused the condition. This can be problematic, since sometimes identifying the cause of a condition is part of the process of finding an appropriate treatment.

Just looking at one or several blood test markers may not provide the doctor with enough information about the ailment or treatment. Blood test results that are high or low may be a normal response for some people.

CHAPTER 11

Foods that strengthen the immune system

Food	Component	What it does
Sauerkraut, kimchi, kefir	D-phenyllactic acid	signals monocytesto to bind to a receptor protein on a cell's surface
Garlic	sulfur compound called allicin	spurs production of macrophages and lymphocytes
Sleep	hurns out integrins	integrands are proteins that help T-cells attach to germ infected cells and destroy them
Cherries		reduce inflammation
Tomatoes, watermellon, Grapefruit, asparagus, mango Red cabbage, carrots	ycopine phytonutrient Contains B-6 & C	One of the Most Powerful Antioxidants in the World. Helps- to Prevent Lycopene plays a role in preventing cancer & promoting Healthy eyes Contains citrulline converts to arginine to create nitric oxide That has benefits on the heart and blood vessels and carry more oxygen May help your eyesight: Lycopene may prevent or delay the formation of cataracts and reduce your risk of macular.degeneration..May reduce pain Lycopene may help reduce neuropathic pain, a type of pain caused by nerve Lycopene can protect your DNA, your prostate health,your skin and your bones and prevent. . Neurological Disorder. .Prevents Stroke & inhibits the development of blood clots that result in a stroke, prevents damage from pesticides, protects the liver, protects against yeast ininfection infection, slows cancer growth, citrulline prevents accumulation of Fat in fat cells

Cayenne	capsicum	has some digestive benefits worth considering. Capsaicin may be able to stimulate digestion and regulate build up of digestive fluids
Apples	quercetin	antioxidant
Blue berries & blackberries Brussells sprouts	Vitamin K	Prevents osteoporosis and hardening of the arteries, antioxidant
Cantelope	betacarotiune & vitamin C	
Pineapple	bromelain, boswellian	reduces inflammation

Bernardio La Palio was 114 years old in 13 August 2015. He owed his longevity to five foods: garlic, chocolate, cinnamon, olive oil and honey. He wasd introduced by Dr. Amy Lee, Bariatric Physician at the Integrative Digestion Center in Las Angeles. Avoid foods with fructose corn syrup found in fruit bars, yogurt, and cereal bars.

Cinnamon	bark of a tree	Reduces body inflammation controlling blood sugar Encourage normal insulin activity Tame sugar cravings, Make you feel fuller after a meal Prevent chronic insulin resistance brought on by a high-sugar diet Prevent long-term damage to tissues due to chronic high blood sugar and insulin resistance Reduce system inflammation, which is the root cause of most chronic diseases

Cayenne	capsaicin Vitamins C, A, & K	lowers blood pressure, digestive health. Forstalls blood clots, Improves strength of veins, digestive health, pain relief on skin,
Bananas	magnesium and potassium	lowers blood pressure reduces bone loss and kidney stones
Asparagus Apricots	Vitamin A &C, folic acid Vitamins A &C, lycopene	linked to cancer prevention in men
Cod liver oil	Vitamin D	promotes calcium absorption & cures rickets
Cranberry juice	Vitamin C	prevent urinary tract infections, reduces cperiodontitis
Kale	Vitamin K, lutein	reduces arthritis
Kidney beans	fiber, iron, protein, potassium, Magnesium, & foliate	
Peanut butter	protein & niacin	
Oranges Prunes	Vitamin C, potassium fiber, potassium, Vitamin A Vitamin B-6, antioxidants	
Brown rice	phosphorus & potassium	

Sweet potatoes	beta-carotene, vitamin, folate Calcium, manganese	
Barley, buckwheat, kasha Quinoa	protects against heart disease, cancer, diabetes	
Yogurt, cheese, milk, tofu	calcium, magnesium, vitamin-12 probiotics aid in digestion	
Sardine, salmon quinoa	omega 3 Vitamin D & calcium	
Shredded wheat	magnesium	reduced risk of diabetes
Spinach	vitamin A & K, folate	reduced risk of macular degeneration
Strawberries Watermelon	anthocyanins, vitamin C vitamin C & A	powerful antioxidant
Processed cheese	contains diacetyl C4H602 provides a buttery or creamy flavor found in many foods	product of fermentation linked to memory loss, lung disease, bronchiolis obliterans

selenium foods eggs, brazil nuts, fish sunflower seeds, turkey chicken breasts, chia seeds, mushrooms	mineral	deficiency: muscle weakness, fatigue, brain fog, thyroid, hair loss, skin and nail discoloration
Almonds	potassium, vitamin E, zxinc riboflavin, & magnesium	
acorn squash	lycopene, folate, potassium, vitamin A& C	
Light tuna, brown rice	niacin (B-3)	deficiency: tiredness, lack of energy and motivation, migraines
Whole wheat bread broccoli	phosphorus	deficiency starvation and is almost never the result of low dietary intakes . nut pread, Phosphorus deficiency (hypophosphatemia) is rare in the United States The effects of hypophosphatemia can include anorexia, anemia, proximal muscle weakness, skeletal effects (bone pain, rickets, and osteomalacia), increased infection risk, paresthesias, ataxia, and confusion

Tumeric & ginger Usually a powder Source Dr.s Marc: Micozzi & Russell Blaylock Red & white wine	belongs to zingiberaceae family helps body achieve homeostasis curcumin is extracted from turmeric contain polyphenols also found in coffee, olive oil and chocolate, red wine contains more polyphenols than white wine	health benefits: Alzheimer's disease, dementia, cancer, depression, pain, gastrointestinal disturbances, heart disease, type II diabetes, slashed fatigue, cuts time for muscle recovery, reduces inflammation Reduced risk of developing: blood clots, brain diseases, cancer, heart, disease, obesity, high blood pressure, high blood sugar

Vitamins and minerals are essential substances that our bodies need to develop and function normally. The known vitamins include A, C, D, E, and K, and the B vitamins: thiamin (B1), riboflavin (B2), niacin (B3), pantothenic acid (B5), pyridoxal (B6), cobalamin (B12), biotin, and folate/folic acid B9. A number of minerals are essential for health: calcium, phosphorus, potassium, sodium, chloride, magnesium, iron, zinc, iodine, sulfur, cobalt, copper, fluoride, manganese, and selenium. The Dietary Guidelines for Americans 2015–2020 recommends that people should aim to meet their nutrient requirements through a healthy eating pattern that includes nutrient-dense forms of food.

Turmeric (zingiberaceae) benefits: arthritis, cancer, depression, GI disturbances, type II diabetes, reduces inflammation, fatigue.

Saw Palmetto berries Bilberries Other names huckleberry Whortleberry , blueberry	maintains healthy prostate and urinary tract, boosts nutrient assimilation improves integrity of capillary walls, anti-clotting, lowers blood sugar, used during WW II to improve night vision by RAF pilots flying at night, improves blood supply to nervous system, collagen rich in Vitamin A and C analgesic properties release of vasodilators, stimulates production of collagen antioxidant that scavenges free radicals, protects macula From degeneration reduces cellular leakage and hemorrhage in the retina, bilberry and vitamin E halts progression of cataracts, improves vision in people with myopia, night blindness, and Glaucoma lowers blood sugar for diabetics.
Coffee (Dr. Marc Micozzi), PhD	lowers risk of skin cancer, colon cancer, cardiovascular disease, & brain disease
Green vegetables, spinach Broccoli, kale, peppers, winter Squash, egg yolks,, collard greens	lutein, zeaxanthin results in less chance of developing cataracts, itb is a yellow crystalline carotenoid alcohol C40H56O2 that is isomeric with lutein and occurs especially in fruits and vegetables
Garlic Vitamins B, B & C Onions Vitamins B, B-6, B-9, C, A	manganese, selenium, iron, copper, potassium, allicin prevent some cancers, lowers blood sugar & cholesterol pyridoxine, manganese, copper
Honey Vitamins C, K, E, B2, B3, B5, B6	Natural honey without maple syrap or sugar added
Avoiding fruits and vegetables Union of Concerned scientists Institute for Nutrition Research In Australia	sore muscles, scurvy, heart disease, diabetes
Piperine	Piperine, along with its isomer chavicine, is the alkaloid responsible for the pungency of black pepper and long pepper. It has een used in some forms of traditional medicine.- increases absorbtion of magnesium, quercettin & curcumin

Dr. Amy Lee, bariatric physician, says the most important foods are: garlic, chocolate, cinnamon, olive oil & honey

Sun exposure

Source: Marc S. Micozzi, M.D., Ph.D.) Intrinsic Photosensitivity Enhances Motility of T Lymphocytes," Scientific Reports 12/20/2016; 6: 3 39479 New evidence out of Georgetown University suggests that sun exposure — even in the dead of winter — can help you fight off colds better and faster. When we talk about sun exposure, most people think about ultraviolet B (UVB) wavelengths. UVB wavelengths are invisible to the human eye. and they also activate vitamin D production in the skin. (And as you know, vitamin D helps fight virtually every disease, including infections.) So most of the research on sun exposure has focused on the UVB ray-vitamin D connection. But for this study, researchers studied a different part of the spectrum — the blue light found in the sun's rays. Blue light comes from the visible spectrum of solar radiation, and it had been studied in Europe for its healing effects.

The Georgetown researchers found that blue light of the sun reaches through the top layer of skin and activates T-cells in your immune system, telling them to move throughout the body. (T-cells help kill microbes. And they reach the site of infection by circulating through the blood. Interestingly, the skin hosts approximately twice as many T-cells as found normally circulating in blood. There is a strong connection between the skin organ and the development of the immune system.) Blue light from the sun increases synthesis of hydrogen peroxide. This synthesis then activates a signaling pathway, increasing T-cell movements. White blood cells in your immune system also release hydrogen peroxide when they come into contact with a microbe to kill it. The release of hydrogen peroxide "calls" more T-cells and other immune cells to recruit them to the site of infection to mount a full immune response. Furthermore, UVB rays that activate vitamin D only penetrate the atmosphere when the sun is high enough, from April through October, in most parts of the U.S.

By comparison, blue light reaches the Earth whenever the sun is shining — 12 months of the year. So you can get your infection-fighting blue light rays year-round by going out in the sun. Maybe the cold and flu season has something to do with not getting enough of the sun's blue rays on your skin during the winter?

Weakening the Immune System Stress Accelerates Immune Aging, Study Finds

June 13, 2022 — Stress -- in the form of traumatic events, job strain, everyday stressors and discrimination -- accelerates aging of the immune system, potentially increasing a person's risk of cancer Immune System News Follow all of Science Daily's **latest research news** and **top science headlines!** June 18, 2022

Chronic stress puts your health at risk

Chronic stress can wreak havoc on your mind and body. Take steps to control your stress.
By Mayo Clinic Staff

Your body is hard-wired to react to stress in ways meant to protect you against threats from predators and other aggressors. Such threats are rare today, but that doesn't mean that life is free of stress.

On the contrary, you likely face many demands each day, such as taking on a huge workload, paying the bills and taking care of your family. Your body treats these so-called minor hassles as threats. As a result, you may feel as if you're constantly under attack. But you can fight back. You don't have to let stress control your life.

Understanding the natural stress response

When you encounter a perceived threat — such as a large dog barking at you during your morning walk — your hypothalamus, a tiny region at your brain's base, sets off an alarm system in your body. Through a combination of nerve and hormonal signals, this system prompts your adrenal glands, located atop your kidneys, to release a surge of hormones, including adrenaline and cortisol.

Adrenaline increases your heart rate, elevates your blood pressure and boosts energy supplies. Cortisol, the primary stress hormone, increases sugars (glucose) in the bloodstream, enhances your brain's use of glucose and increases the availability of substances that repair tissues.

Cortisol also curbs functions that would be nonessential or harmful in a fight-or-flight situation. It alters immune system responses and suppresses the digestive system, the reproductive system and growth processes. This complex natural alarm system also communicates with the brain regions that control mood, motivation and fear.

Stress and Isolation can Effect Your Physical Health

Mental health conditions often elicit a psychological response. Research suggests that people who feel more politically different than the average voters in their state experience more days of poor physical health each month . Fearing people with opposing viewpoints causes a constant state of "arousal and anxiety." Stress causes the brain to release the chemical cortisol , which regulates your body's response to stress. Dr.Michaek Roeke Psy.D, (Senior Director of the Center for Research and Innovation at Newport Health Care) says that moderate stress can actually be good for you, especially if you're "impassioned by it and it is not preoccupying.

Too much cortisol long-term can impact the immune system, and cause muscle weakness, high blood pressure, high blood sugar, and obesity. Chronic stress can make you irritable and cause conditions, like heart attack, strokes, and chronic pain. Dr. MichaeklRoeke said "We are not set up for this constant onslaught of stress around the political divisiveness that is happening now.

When the natural stress response goes wild

The body's stress response system is usually self-limiting. Once a perceived threat has passed, hormone levels return to normal. As adrenaline and cortisol levels drop, your heart rate and blood pressure return to baseline levels, and other systems resume their regular activities. But when stressors are always present and you constantly feel under attack, that fight-or-flight reaction stays turned on.The long-term activation of the stress response system and the overexposure to cortisol and other stress hormones that follows can disrupt almost all your body's processes. This puts you at increased risk of many health problems, including:

- Anxiety
- Depression
- Digestive problems
- Headaches
- Muscle tension and pain
- Heart disease, heart attack, high blood pressure and stroke
- Sleep problems
- Weight gain
- Memory and concentration impairment

That's why it's so important to learn healthy ways to cope with your life stressors.

Why you react to life stressors the way you do

Your reaction to a potentially stressful event is different from anyone else's. How you react to your life stressors is affected by such factors as:

- **Genetics.** The genes that control the stress response keep most people on a fairly steady emotional level, only occasionally priming the body for fight or flight. Overactive or underactive stress responses may stem from slight differences in these genes.
- **Life experiences.** Strong stress reactions sometimes can be traced to traumatic events. People who were neglected or abused as children tend to be particularly vulnerable to stress. The same is true of airplane crash survivors, military personnel, police officers and firefighters, and people who have experienced violent crime.

You may have some friends who seem relaxed about almost everything and others who react strongly to the slightest stress. Most people react to life stressors somewhere between those extremes.

Learning to react to stress in a healthy way

Stressful events are facts of life. And you may not be able to change your current situation. But you can take steps to manage the impact these events have on you. You can learn to identify what causes you stress and how to take care of yourself physically and emotionally in the face of stressful situations.

Stress management strategies include:

Eating a healthy diet, getting regular exercise and getting plenty of sleep

- Practicing relaxation techniques such as yoga, deep breathing, massage or meditation
- Keeping a journal and writing about your thoughts or what you're grateful for in your life
- Taking time for hobbies, such as reading, listening to music, or watching your favorite show or movie

- Fostering healthy friendships and talking with friends and family
- Having a sense of humor and finding ways to include humor and laughter in your life, such as watching funny movies or looking at joke websites
- Volunteering in your community
- Organizing and prioritizing what you need to accomplish at home and work and removing tasks that aren't necessary
- Seeking professional counseling, which can help you develop specific coping strategies to manage stress

Avoid unhealthy ways of managing your stress, such as using alcohol, tobacco, drugs or excess food. If you're concerned that your use of these products has increased or changed due to stress, talk to your doctor.

The rewards for learning to manage stress can include peace of mind, less stress and anxiety, a better quality of life, improvement in conditions such as high blood pressure, better self-control and focus, and better relationships. And it might even lead to a longer, healthier life.

CHAPTER 12

Representative Chemical Composition of Urine

Water % H2O	95	%
Urea (H2NCONH2)	9.3 - 23.3	g/l
Chloride(Cl)	1.87 - 8.4	g/l
Sodium (Na)	1.17 - 4.39	g/l
Potassium (K)	0.750 - 2.61	g/l
Inorganic sulfur (S)	0.163 - 1.80	g/l
Creatinine (C4H7N3O)	0.670 - 2.15	g/l

Ketones produced by liver when cells do not get enough glucose, complicates diabetes, called ketonuria Protein in urine from dehydration, proteinuria high stress, fever, being in a cold temperature,, kidney problem

CHAPTER 13

Essential Minerals that the Body Needs

An essential mineral is any mineral required by the body for health, that cannot be produced by the body and so has to be provided by your diet. There are 21 essential minerals, often described as:

List of 5 major minerals (a.k.a. electrolytes)
The five major minerals in your body are also classified as electrolytes.

They form chemistry reactions when mixed with water, moving in and out of your cells to help keep your body hydrated, ensures your nerves and muscles are functioning properly, balances your blood pH and maintains your blood pressure, among their many functions.

- calcium
- phosphorus
- potassium
- sodium
- magnesium

CHAPTER 14

List of 16 Trace Minerals (a.k.a. micro minerals)

Trace minerals are also known as micro minerals as the human body only needs them in much smaller amounts, although that doesn't mean that they are less important.
Among the minerals in this list, iron is a major component of your red blood cells. Its main function is to help carry oxygen and nutrients to be distributed to your entire body.

- iron
- zinc
- cobalt
- copper
- manganese
- molybdenum
- iodine
- selenium
- sulfur
- chloride
- boron
- silicon
- vanadium
- nickel
- arsenic
- chromium

CHAPTER 15

Essential Minerals List and their Roles in the Body

First off, it's important to note that no mineral is used in isolation by the body. All minerals interact with other minerals, vitamins, enzymes etc. For example, it is overly simplistic to say calcium makes healthy bones, as magnesium and phosphorus must also be present to build bones.

The following five major essential minerals are found in the largest amounts in a human body:

1. Calcium (*Ca*)
Found in teeth, bones and nails: Calcium is the most abundant mineral in the body. Roles of calcium in the body: Calcium is essential for the clotting of blood, the action of certain enzymes and the control of the passage of fluids through the cell walls. It is also essential to normal heart action and muscle contraction. Symptoms of calcium deficiency: Weaker bones, delayed growth, nervous irritability and muscle sensitivity. Good sources of calcium: Green leafy vegetables such as broccoli and cabbage, seeds, nuts, dates, oranges and tofu. Though high in calcium, dairy products are acid-forming so they are not a good source.

2. Phosphorus (*P*)
Phosphorus is found in bones, teeth, and the protoplasm and nucleus of every cell. It is used in more bodily functions than any other mineral. Roles of phosphorus in the body: Phosphorus is used to build healthy bones and teeth (in combination with calcium); to metabolize carbohydrates, fats and proteins; to build nerve and brain cells. Symptoms of phosphorus deficiency: Poor bone and teeth development, mental fatigue, feeling of depression resulting from exhausted nerve energy. Good sources of phosphorus: Coconut, green leafy vegetables, pears, apple, avocado, dates, carrots, rice, oats, fish, legumes.

3. Potassium (*K*)

Roles of potassium in the body: Potassium regulates transportation in and out of cells including the removal of toxins and delivery of nutrients, regulates the heart beat, tissue elasticity, aids healing, promotes correct liver functioning and regulates nerve and muscle action. Symptoms of potassium deficiency: Poor muscular control, poor digestion, liver problems, slow healing of sores. Good sources of potassium: Cereals, most fresh fruit and vegetables, bananas, papaya, fish, pulses, nuts and seeds.

4. Sodium (*Na*)

Roles of sodium in the body: With potassium, sodium regulates exchange in and out of cells; helps maintain water balance; is required to produce digestive juices; helps eliminate carbon dioxide; aids correct nerve functioning. Symptoms of sodium deficiency: Muscle cramp, nausea, indigestion, arthritis, rheumatism, gallbladder and kidney stones. Good sources of sodium: Seeds, strawberry, melon, sea asparagus, fish, natural extracted salts. Note that sodium chloride (refined table salt) is a bad source of sodium and poisonous to the body.

5. Magnesium (*Mg*)

Roles of magnesium in the body: Required for more than 300 biochemical reactions, maintain normal nerve and muscle function, supports a healthy immune system, carbohydrate metabolism. Symptoms of magnesium deficiency: Poor complexion, faster heartbeat, irritability, digestive disorders, soft bones. asthma, restless leg syndrome, muscle cramps and spasms, stress, depression and anxiety, sleep problems, high blood pressures, ringing in ears, cardio vascular problems, osteroporosis, low energy, leg cramps (take magnesium gluconate for nocturnal cramps)

Good sources of magnesium: Nuts (especially walnut and almonds), cereals, spinach, fish.figs, dark chocolate, whole grains, figs, soybeans, wild rice, dried oriander, fatty fish, salmon, tuna, tofu, yogurt, kefir, chickpeas, lentils, bananas, leafy greens, flaxseed oil, dates, oatmeal, coffee,

Symptoms of Excess Magnesium diarrhea, nausea, stomach upset, abdominal cramps, vomiting, hypotension (rapid decrease in blood pressure), erratic heart rhythms,, slow heart beat, breathing difficulty, muscle weakness, confusion & lethargy,

List of 16 Trace Minerals Required by the Human Body

As the name implies, trace minerals are required in far smaller amounts (less than 100 mg/day). Each has a specific biochemical function in the human body. They are needed in such tiny amounts that the role of many were not discovered until recently, and the essentiality of some is still being debated.

1. Iron (*Fe*)
Iron is best known for its role as a primary constituent of haemoglobin in red blood cells. Roles of iron in the body: Transportation of oxygen and carbon dioxide around the body; building of bones and muscle tissue. Symptoms of iron deficiency: Pale complexion, anemia, low energy levels, stunted growth. Good sources of iron: Dark green vegetables, legumes, dried fruits, whole grain cereals, spinach, liver. **Excess iron**; may cause liver cancer

2. Manganese (*Mn*)
Manganese is found in the liver, kidneys, pancreas, lungs, prostrate, adrenal gland, brain and bones. Roles of manganese in the body: Facilitates chemical reactions, carbohydrate metabolism, strong tissues and bone, helps form thyroxine, helps regulate blood sugar levels, needed for antioxidant and enzyme function. Symptoms of manganese deficiency: Weak bones, anemia, chronic fatigue, low immunity, hormonal imbalance, infertility. Good sources of manganese: Beans, walnut, whole cereals, green vegetables, cabbage, sweet potato.

3. Copper (*Cu*)
Copper is found in the heart, lungs, liver and gallbladder. Roles of copper in the body: Copper is required primarily for the absorption and metabolism of iron. Symptoms of copper deficiency: Copper deficiency symptoms are similar to those of iron: poor hemoglobin production, pale complexion, anemia, low energy levels, stunted growth, hypercupremia, fatigue, headaches, nausea, moodiness, depression, ittitability Good sources of copper: Nuts and seeds, raisins, shellfish.

4. **Iodine (*I*)**
Found mainly in the thyroid gland in the throat. Roles of iodine in the body: Used to make thyroxine which regulates some of the metabolic functions; oxidation of fats and proteins. Symptoms of iodine deficiency: Swollen thyroid gland, goiter, low metabolism. Good sources of iodine: Nuts and seeds, raisins, green leafy vegetables, turnip, banana, watermelon, shellfish, seaweeds, sea salt, fish, whole cereals and grains.

5. Zinc (*Zn*)

Roles of zinc in the body: Regulation of blood sugar, healing of wounds, transfer of carbon dioxide from tissue to lungs.Symptoms of zinc deficiency: Poor intestinal absorption, restricted growth, prostrate problems, absence of taste. Good sources of zinc: Nuts and seeds, shellfish, cereal products such as wheat germ. Though they contain zinc, dairy products are acid-forming so not a good source. Excessive zinc Signs: Nausea. Nausea is a common side effect when potent zinc supplements are consumed in excess to treat a cold or in some... Stomach Pain. Stomach pain is a comorbid symptom of zinc overdose that often occurs with nausea, vomiting, and diarrhea. Fever & Chills....

6. Cobalt (*Co*)

Roles of cobalt in the body: Cobalt helps treat illnesses such as anemia and some infectious diseases; absorption and processing of vitamin B12; aids in repair of myelin, which surrounds and protects nerve cells; helps in the formation of hemoglobin in red blood cells. Symptoms of cobalt deficiency: Anemia, decreased nerve function. Good sources of cobalt: Shiitake mushrooms, fish, shellfish, nuts, legumes, spinach, turnip, figs.

7. Molybdenum (*Mo*)

Many people have probably never heard of molybdenum, required in tiny quantities in the body, it is crucial to good health. Roles of molybdenum in the body: Promotes normal cell function, facilitates waste removal, acts as a catalyst for enzymes, facilitates the breakdown of some amino acids, supports the production of red blood cells. Symptoms of molybdenum deficiency: As molybdenum deficiency in humans is extremely rare, symptoms are not well established. Good sources of molybdenum : Legumes, whole grains, nuts.

8. **Selenium (*Se*)**

Roles of selenium in the body: Supports the immune system; acts as a powerful antioxidant that fights free-radicals, especially when combined with vitamin E. Antioxidants such as selenium help fight damaging particles in the body known as free radicals, protects the thyroid, converts T4 into T3, improves asthma, repairs DNA, increases testtoserone Symptoms of selenium deficiency: Free radicals can damage cell membranes and DNA, adversely affect health and may cause premature ageing

Weight loss, loss of hair, poor digestion, anemia, hypothyroidism

Good sources of selenium: Brazil nuts, seeds, fish, green vegetables.

9. Sulfur (S)

Sulfur is found in the hair, nails, cartilage and blood. Roles of sulfur in the body: Sulfur aids digestion, waste elimination, bile secretion, purification of the system. Symptoms of sulfur deficiency: Restricted growth, eczema, unhealthy nails and hair. Good sources of sulfur: Cabbage, onions, garlic, leeks, avocado, strawberry, cucumber, peach.

10. Chloride (*Cl-*)

Chloride is a negatively charged ion in the blood, where it represents 70% of the body's total negative ion content. Roles of chloride in the body: Functions as an electrolyte; forms hydrochloric acid, a powerful digestive enzyme; aids digestion of metallic minerals; aids absorption of vitamin B12; helps maintain electrical neutrality across the stomach membrane; helps regulate blood pH and transport of carbon dioxide; promotes normal heart activity; aids the transport of electrical impulses throughout the body. Symptoms of chloride deficiency: Overly alkaline blood leading to alkalosis, which is life-threatening; poor digestion; waste retention. Good sources of chloride: Seaweeds, naturally extracted salt, olives, rye, tomato, celery.

11. Boron(*B*)

Roles of boron in the body: Boosts bone density, activates vitamin D, effects how the body handles other minerals, boosts estrogen levels in older women. Symptoms of boron deficiency: Arthritis, weak bones and osteoporosis, weaker muscles, poor concentration and memory loss, premature skin ageing, orsened menopausal and PMS symptoms, allergies. Good sources of boron: Plant-based foods including nuts, legumes, chickpeas, most vegetables, bananas, avocado, broccoli, oranges, red grapes, apples, pears.

12. Silicon (*Si*)

Silicon is found in the pancreas, blood, muscles, skin, nerves, nails, hair, connective tissue and teeth. Roles of silicon in the body: Strong bones, promotes firmness and strength in the tissues, forms part of the arteries, tendons, skin, connective tissue, and eyes. Collagen contains silicon, essentially holding the body tissues together. Symptoms of silicon deficiency: Premature graying or baldness, skin irritations and rashes, possible tooth decay. Good sources of silicon: Red wine, raisins, whole grains, bran, green beans, bananas, root vegetables, spinach, seafood.

13. Vanadium (*Va*)
Vanadium was named after the Scandinavian goddess of beauty, youth, and luster. Roles of vanadium in the body: Regulation of sodium, the metabolism of glucose and lipids, aids the production of red blood cells, encourages normal tissue growth, reduces high blood sugar by mimicking the effects of insulin. Symptoms of vanadium deficiency: May contribute to high cholesterol and irregular blood sugar levels leading to diabetes or hypoglycemia.ood sources of vanadium: Safflower, seeds, corn, parsley, dill, green beans, carrots, cabbage, garlic, tomatoes, radishes and onions. Cooking oils such as olive, sunflower and peanut oils also contain vanadium.

14. Nickel (*Ni*)
Nickel is present in DNA and RNA which means it is found in every cell of the human body. Roles of nickel in the body: Plays a major role in helping the body absorb iron; helps prevent anemia; strengthens bones. Symptoms of nickel deficiency: Infection of the urinary tract; severe allergic reactions (usually skin rashes), anemia, hormonal imbalance, abnormal bone growth, impaired Liver function. Good sources of nickel: Fish, most nuts and seeds, cocoa, alfalfa seeds, oatmeal.

15. Arsenate (*As*)
Important note: Organically-bound arsenic (or arsenate) and elemental arsenic are an essential mineral that comes from plants and animals and are not toxic. In fact, they are handled fairly easily by the body and eliminated by the kidneys. Inorganic arsenic is toxic to humans. Roles of arsenate in the body: The biological function is not fully understood—though arsenic may have a roll in correct cardiac functioning. Symptoms of arsenate deficiency: Unknown. Good sources of arsenate: Seeds and nuts, grains, fruit, vegetables.

16. Chromium (*Cr*)
Chromium is a metallic element required in trace amounts. Roles of chromium in the body: Regulates blood sugar; plays a role in metabolism of carbohydrates, fats, and proteins. Symptoms of chromium deficiency: Fluctuating blood glucose level, fatigue, weaker bones and bone loss, high cholesterol levels, loss of concentration, poor memory. Good sources of chromium: Whole grains, grapes, broccoli, mushrooms, fish, potato
Homocysteine: Levels, Tests, High Homocysteine Levels

Homocysteine is an amino acid. Vitamins B12, B6 and folate break down homocysteine to create other chemicals your body needs. high homocysteine levels have a vitamin deficiency. Without treatment, elevated homocysteine increases your risks for dementia,

heart disease and stole may mean you have omocysteine is an amino acid produced by the body by chemically altering adenosine. Amino acids are naturally made products, which are the building blocks of all the proteins in the body. Most labs report normal ranges of homocysteine as about 4-15 μml/L. Can elevated homocysteine levels be genetic?

Homocysteine is a type of amino acid, a chemical your body uses to make proteins. Normally, vitamin B12, vitamin B6, and folic acid break down homocysteine and change it into other substances your body needs. There should be very little homocysteine left in the bloodstream, < 9 micromols/Liter is recommended. Homocysteine is a type of amino acid. Your body naturally makes it. But at high levels, it can damage the lining of arteries. It can encourage blood clotting. This may raise your risk for coronary artery disease, heart attacks, blood clots, and strokes. High levels of homocysteine may be cause by low levels of: Vitamin B-12

CHAPTER 16

Normal Ranges of Blood Components (F is for females)

Blood Component		Desired Range Internet	Desired Range Enzo Labs	Desired Range Quest Diagnostics	Nursing Reference Guide	Dimensions
A1c Glucose Control for Diabetes %			< 5.7			Percent
A1c Glucose Risk of Diabetes			5.7 – 6.4			Percent
A1c Glucose consistent with diabetes			> 6.5			Percent
Absolute Neutrophils		1500 – 7800	1650-8500	1500-7800		Cells/mL
Absolute Lymphocytes		850-3900	1000-3850	850-3900		Cells/mL
Absolute Lymphocytes	F			1500-7800		Cells/microliter
Absolute Monocytes		200-950	30-850	200-950		Cells.mL
Absolute Monocytes	F			850-3900		Cells/microliter
Absolute Eosinophils		15-500	0-600	15-500		Cells/mL
Absolute Eosinophils	F			200-950		Cells/microliter
Absolute Basophils		0-200	0-120	0-200		Cells/mL
Absolute Basophils	F			15-500		Cells/microliter
Absolute Immature Granulocyte			<91			10E3/microL
Albumin/Globulin Ratio			UNK	1.0-2.5		Ratio
Albumin/Globulin Ratio	F			1.9-3.7		Grams/dL

Blood Component		Desired Range Internet	Desired Range Enzo Labs	Desired Range Quest Diagnostics	Nursing Reference Guide	Dimensions
AST (SGOT) liver function		10.0-35.00	0-40	10-35	10-34	Units/Liter
AST	F				37-153	Units/Liter
ALT (SGPT) alcohol test		9.00-60.00	0-41	9-46	7-56	Units/Liter
ALT	F				10-35	Units/Liter
Alkaline Phosphatase			40-129	40-115	44-147	Units/Liter
Alkaline Phosphatase	F			0.2-1.2		Milligrams/dL
Acid (Folate) Vitamin B-12			> 4.0			Nanograms/mL
Antibodies for SARS Covid 19	F			>1		Antibodies present
Antibodies for SARS Covid 19				>1		Antibodies present
Basophils %			0-2	0-2		Percent
Basophils %	F			0-8		Percent
Bilirubin, Total			0.0-1.2	0.2-1.2	0.3-1.9	Milligrams/dL
Bilirubin, Total	F				1.0-2.5	Milligrams/dL
BUN/Creatine Ratio				6-22	6-20	Ratio
BUN/Creatine Ratio	F			>60		Millilirers/min
BUN Urea Nitrogen	F			<5.7%		Percent
BUN urea nitrogen in blood		7.00-25.00			6-20	Milligrams/dL
BUN	F				6-29	Units/Liter
B Lymphocytes %					4-16	Percent
Carbon Dioxide		21-33	21-32	20-31		Micrimoles/
Carbon Dioxide	F			98-110		Nmol/L
Calcium		8.6-10.2	8.6-10.4	8.6-10.3	8.5-10.2	Micromoles/
Calcium	F			0-32		Nmol/L

Blood Component		Desired Range Internet	Desired Range Enzo Labs	Desired Range Quest Diagnostics	Nursing Reference Guide	Dimensions
Chloride		98-110	98-107	98-110		
Chloride	F			3.5-5.3	3.7-5.2	Nmol/L
Cholestrerol (desired)			<200	<200	<200	Mg/dL
Cholesterol Borderline High			200-239			Mg/dL
Cholesterol HIgh			>240			Mg/dL
Cholesterol/HDL Ratio Desirable			<4.80	<5.0		Ratio
Copper desired <150		71-180				Micrograms/dL
Cortisol (morning)		10-20				Micrograms/dL
Cortisol (evening)		3-10				Micrograms/dL
Creatnine		0.76-1.46	0.7-1.3	0.70-1.11	0.6-1.3	Milligrams/dL
Creatnine	F			7-25		Milligrams/dL
Creatine Kinase, Total	F			29-143		Units/Liter
C-reactive protein		<1				Mg/L
Cytokines (see below)		<1.0				Picograms/milliliter
eGFR			>=60			mL/min.1.73m
Eosinophils %			0-6	0-8		Percent
Eosinophils %	F			0-13		Percent
Glucose	F				65-99	Milligrams/dL
Glucose Fasting		65-99	65-140	65-99	72-100	Mg/dL
Globulin		2.1-3.7	UNK	1.9-3.7		Grams/dL
Globulin	F			3.6-5.1		Grams/dL
HDL Cholesterol Low			>40			Mg/dL
HDL Cholesterol Desired			>60	>40	40-60	Mg/dL
Hematocrit %		38.5-50.0	38.8-50.0	38.5-50.0	42-52	Percent
Hematocrit	F			11.7-15.5		Grams/dL

Blood Component		Desired Range Internet	Desired Range Enzo Labs	Desired Range Quest Diagnostics	Nursing Reference Guide	Dimensions
Hemoglobin		13.2-17.1	13.5-17.5	13.2-17.1	12-8	Grams/dL
Hemoglobin	F			3.80-5.10		Million/microliter
Hemoglobin A1c% of Hgb			4.1-5.6	<5.7		Percent
Hypoglycemia		<70mg/dcl				Mg/dL
Hyperglycemia		>200mg/dcl				Mg/dL
If O 2<90% (see doctor)						Percent
Immature Granulocytes %			<1			Percent
Iron Ferritin		30-400	30-170			Micrograms/dL
Keytones (see below)		=<20				G/dL
LDL Cholesterol Desired			<100	<100		Mg/dL
LDL Cholesterol Above Optimal			100-129			Mg/dL
LDL Cholesterol Borderline High			130-159			Mg/dL
LDL Cholesterol High			160-189			Mg/dL
LDL Cholesterol Very High			>190			Mg/dL
Lead (from drinking water) NIOSH		<50				Micrograms/dL
Lead (from drinking water) children		<5				Micrograms/dL
Leukocyte Esterase (see below)		<1+(75 Leu/L)				Leu/microliter
Lymphocytes %			15.0-46.0	15-49		Percent
Lymphocytes %			15.0-46.0	15-49		Percent
Lymphocytes %	F			38-80		Percent
Magnesium		2.75-4.80		1.5-2.5		Milligrams/dL
Magnesium	F			1.5-2.5		Milligrams/dL
Mercury (from fish) Nat'lAcad. Of Sci.		<85				Micrograms/liter
Mercury (from fish) EPA Reference		<5.8				Micrograms/liter

Blood Component		Desired Range Internet	Desired Range Enzo Labs	Desired Range Quest Diagnostics	Nursing Reference Guide	Dimensions
MCV		80-100	82-100	80-100	78-100	fL
MCV %				35.0-45.0		Percent
MCH		27-33	26-34	27-33	27-31	Picograms
MCH	F			80.0-100.0		Ft
MCHC		32-36	32-36	32.0-36.0	33-37	G/dL
MCHC	F			27.0-33.0		Picograms
Monocytes %			2.0-14.0	0-13		percent
Monocytes %	F			15-49		percent
MPV			7.0-13.0	7.5-12.5		fL
MPV	F			140-400		Thousand/microliter
Neutrophils				0-200		Cells/microliter
Neutrophils %			43.0-77.0	38-80		percent
Neutrophils	F			0-200		Cells/microliter
Non-HDL Cholesterol Desired				<130		Mg/dL
NRBC %			0.0-0.70			Percent/100WBC
NRBC Count			Unknown			Unknown
Oxygen (oximeter)		95-100%				percent
PH				5.0-8.0		No dimension
Platelet Count		140-400	150-450	140-400		10E3/microL
Platelet Count %	F			11.0-15.0		percent
Potassium		3.5-5.3	3.5-5.3	3.5-5.3	3.7-5.2	
Potassium	F			135-146		
Protein		6.2-8.3	6.0-8.3	6.1-8.1		Grams/dL
Protein	F			8.6-10.4		Milligrams/dL
Protein in urine		1-20 is high, normal = <150				Grams/day
Protein in blood		6-8.3				Grams/dL

Blood Component		Desired Range Internet	Desired Range Enzo Labs	Desired Range Quest Diagnostics	Nursing Reference Guide	Dimensions
PSA Prostate Specific Antegen		0-4.0				Nanograms/mL
RDW %		11.6-15.0 b	11.8-15.6	11.0-15.0		percent
RDW	F			32.0-36.0		Grams/dL
Red Blood Cell Count		4.2-5.8	4.2-5.8	4.20-5.80	4.2-5.6	Millioin/mL
Sed Rate ESR				0-20		Mm/hr
Sodium		135-146	136-145	135-146	135-145	Nmol/L
Specific Gravity				1.001-1.035		No dimension
T3 Uptake %				22-35		percent
T3 Total	F			76-181		Nanograms/dL
T3 Uptake %			27-41	22-35		percent
T4 (thyroxine)	F			5.1-11.9		Micrograms/dL Folic
Thyroxine, Total (T4)			4.5-11.7			Micrograms/dL
Thyroxine, Free (FT4)			0.80-1.70			Micrograms/dL
Thyroxine Free T4 Index		0.80-1.70			1.4-3.8	Micrograms/dL
TIBC			225-415			Micrograms/dL
T Lymphocytes %					60-80	percent
Transferrin Saturation %			14-50			percent
Triglycerides Desired			<150	<150	<150	Mg/dL
Triglycerides Borderline High			150-199			Mg/dL
Triglycerides High			200-499			Mg/dL
Triglycerides Very High			>500			Mg/dL
TSH			0.270-4.20	0.40-4.50	0.4-4.5	microIU/mL
TSH	F				0.4-4.50	mLU/Liter
UIBC			112-347			Micrograms/dL

Blood Component	Desired Range Internet	Desired Range Enzo Labs	Desired Range Quest Diagnostics	Nursing Reference Guide	Dimensions
Uric Acid		4.0 – 8.0 > 18 years	4.0 - 8.0		milligrams/dL
Urea Nitrogen		6 - 20	7 - 25		mg/dL
VLDV Cholesterol Calc. Desirable		< 30			mg/dL
Vitamin B-12		232 – 1245			picograms/mL
Vitamin D 1,25		19.9 – 79.3	30 - 100		picograms/mL
White blood cell count	3.8 – 10.8	3.8 – 10.5	3.8 – 10.8	4 – 10.5	housand/mL
Zinc	60 – 130				micrograms/dL

Leukocyte Esterase is an enzyme released by white blood cells in urine, a result of an infection or inflammation The <1 means that the color and gross properties of the uriune test sample are normal.

Ketones in urine test measures ketone levels in your urine. Normally, the cells in your body use glucose (sugar) from your blood for energy. If your cells can't get enough glucose, your body breaks down fat for energy instead. This produces an acid called ketones, which can build up in your blood and urine. Keytones >60 mg/dL indicates complication of diabetes.

Cytokines are small proteins that are crucial in controlling the growth and activity of other immune system cells and blood cells. When released, they signal the immune system to do its job. Cytokines affect the growth of all blood cells and other cells that help the body's immune and inflammation responses. They also help to boost anti-cancer activity by sending signals that can help make abnormal cells die and normal cells live longer. Range of measured cytokines Detection range of cytokines in all tested serum samples from patients with COVID-19 hospitalized at the Mount Sinai Health System (orange, n = 1,959), in comparison with serum samples from healthy donors (black, n = 9) and plasma samples from patients with multiple myeloma prior to (blue, n = 151) and during (red, n = 121) CRS induced by CAR T cell therapy. Heavy bars indicate median, and error bars represent 95% CI, each value indicated by a dot. Pair wise comparisons by the two-sided Mann–Whitney t-test show significantly higher levels of IL-6, IL-8 and TNF-α in COVID-19 samples compared to samples from healthy donors of patients with non-CRS cancer (****P < 0.0001, ***P

< 0.001, **P < 0.01 and *P < 0.05; NS, not significant). Median, mean and range are shown in Extended Data Fig. 1d (error band indicates the median with 95% CI). HD, hemodialysis An inflammatory cytokine signature predicts COVID-19 severity and survival Cytokine Release Syndrome (CRS), Patients with Cytokine level above 1.0 picograms per milliter are immunocompromised. CAR-T means Chimeric Antigen receptors on T Cells. IL-6, IL-8, TNF, and IL1 are different cytokines.

Several studies have revealed that the hyper-inflammatory response induced by severe acute respiratory syndrome coronavirus 2 (SARS-CoV-2) is a major cause of disease severity and death. However, predictive biomarkers of pathogenic inflammation to help guide targetable immune pathways are critically lacking. We implemented a rapid multiplex cytokine assay to measure serum interleukin (IL)-6, IL-8, tumor necrosis factor

Several studies have revealed that the hyper-inflammatory response induced by severe acute respiratory syndrome coronavirus 2 (SARS-CoV-2) is a major cause of disease severity and death. However, predictive biomarkers of pathogenic inflammation to help guide targetable immune pathways are critically lacking. We implemented a rapid multiplex cytokine assay to measure serum interleukin (IL)-6, IL-8, tumor necrosis factor (TNF)-α and IL-1β in hospitalized patients with corona virus disease 2019 (COVID-19) upon admission to the Mount Sinai Health System in New York.

Patients (n = 1,484) were followed up to 41 d after admission (median, 8 d), and clinical information, laboratory test results and patient outcomes were collected. We found that high serum IL-6, IL-8 and TNF-α levels at the time of hospitalization were strong and independent predictors of patient survival ($P < 0.0001$, $P = 0.0205$ and $P = 0.0140$, respectively). Notably, when adjusting for disease severity, common laboratory inflammation markers.

According to Dr. Mark Rosenberg, overactive cytokines imply high stress and this condition is responsible for four of countries top killers: heart disease, Alzheimer's, cancer, and lower respiratory diseases. A high c-reactive protein and the sedimentation rate indicates that the immune system is stressed out.

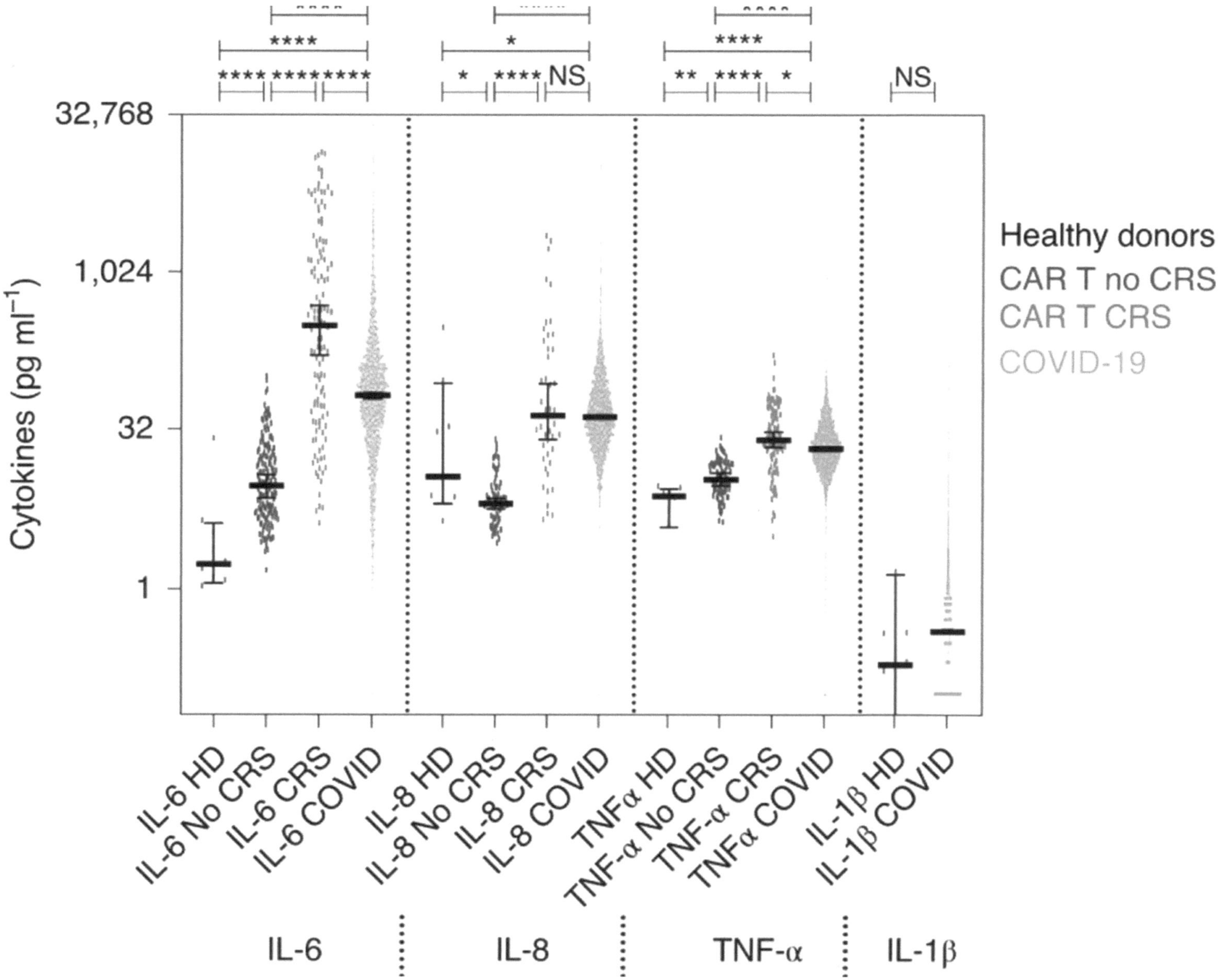

NS
32,768
1,024
32
1
Cytokines (pg ml^{-1})
Healthy donors
CAR T no CRS
CAR T CRS
COVID-19
IL-6 HD
IL-6 No CRS
IL-6 CRS
IL-6 COVID
IL-8 HD
IL-8 No CRS
IL-8 CRS
IL-8 COVID
TNFα HD
TNF-α No CRS
TNF-α CRS
TNFα COVID
IL-1β HD
IL-1β COVID
IL-6
IL-8
TNF-α
IL-1β

Patients (n = 1,484) were followed up to 41 d after admission (median, 8 d), and clinical information, laboratory test results and patient outcomes were collected. We found that high serum IL-6, IL-8 and TNF-α levels at the time of hospitalization were strong and independent predictors of patient survival ($P < 0.0001$, $P = 0.0205$ and $P = 0.0140$, respectively). Notably, when adjusting for disease severity, common laboratory inflammation markers, hypoxia and other vitals, demographics, and a range of co-morbidities, IL-6 and TNF-α serum levels remained independent and significant predictors of disease severity and death. These findings were validated in a second cohort of patients (n = 231). We propose that serum IL-6 and TNF-α levels should be considered in the management and treatment of patients with COVID-19 to stratify prospective clinical trials, guide resource allocation and inform therapeutic options. Elevated levels of serum IL-6 and TNF-α at the time of hospitalization are independent and significant predictors of clinical outcome in two cohorts of patients with COVID-19.

CONCLUSION

I have tried to present useful information to patients who have had a bloold test. I have listed essential minerals and the foods that contain the minerals and the consequence if the minerals are absent. Especially is the role of magnesium because it manages insulin levels to prevent blood sugar spikes, regulates energy levels, muscle and nerve functions, electrical conductivity to contract muscles, and assists to have a steady heart beat all described by Dr. T. H. Chan , of the Harvard School of Public Health.

I presented information about cortisol which is essential for emotional stability and the consequence of having excessive cortisol because it compromises the immune system and has negative consequences for unattended infants.

This booklet may be modified upon development of new results from blood or urine tests for telomeres, ageing and cancer cells. Telomeres are the caps on the ends of chromosomes. Elongated caps are correlated with potential cancer. Recent research has been able to identify cancer cells in blood and urine. So far I found no quantifiable results from research on telomere length and cancer cells in blood or urine.

www.ingramcontent.com/pod-product-compliance
Lightning Source LLC
LaVergne TN
LVHW071513220926
848486LV00009BA/369